CHARLES VAN RIPER, editor *Foundations of Speech Pathology Series*

Prentice-Hall Foundations of Speech Pathology Series

Cluttering

PRENTICE-HALL INTERNATIONAL, INC., *London*
PRENTICE-HALL OF AUSTRALIA, PTY., LTD., *Sydney*
PRENTICE-HALL OF CANADA, LTD., *Toronto*
PRENTICE-HALL OF INDIA (PRIVATE) LTD., *New Delhi*
PRENTICE-HALL OF JAPAN, INC., *Tokyo*
PRENTICE-HALL DE MEXICO, S.A., *Mexico City*

Cluttering

DESO A. WEISS M.D.

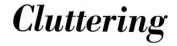

Prentice-Hall, Inc., *Englewood Cliffs, N.J.*

editor's note

THE SET OF VOLUMES WHICH CONSTITUTES THE *Foundations of Speech Pathology Series* is designed to serve as the nucleus of a professional library, both for students of speech pathology and audiology and for the practicing clinician. Each individual text in the series is written by an author whose authority has long been recognized in his field. Each author has done his utmost to provide the basic information concerning the speech or hearing disorders covered in his book. Our new profession needs new tools, good ones, to be used not once but many times. The flood of new information already upon us requires organization if it is to be assimilated and if it is to help us solve the many different professional problems which beset us. This series provides that essential organization.

One of the unifying and outstanding features of all the volumes in this series is the use of search items. In addition to providing the core of information concerning his subject, each author has indicated clearly other sources having significance for the topic being discussed. The reader is urged to explore, to search, and to discover—and the trails are charted. In so rapidly changing a profession as ours, we cannot afford to remain content with what we have been taught. We must learn to continue learning.

Although each individual volume in this series is complete *ix*

unto itself, the instructor should welcome the opportunity presented by the *Foundations of Speech Pathology Series* to combine several volumes to form the basic structure of the course he
teaches. They may also be used as collateral readings. These
short but comprehensive books give the instructor a thoroughly
flexible teaching tool. But the primary aim of the authors of
these texts has been the creation of a basic library for all of our
students and professional workers. In this series we have sought
to provide a common fund of knowledge to help unify and serve
our new profession.   ϑϑϑ

preface

CLUTTERING HAS BEEN DISCUSSED IN THE LITERATURE OF SPEECH pathology for more than two thousand years. Although mentioned at least briefly by almost every nineteenth century encyclopedist in the field,* the first complete volume devoted to cluttering did not appear until 1963,† indicating that cluttering is only now beginning to receive the attention it deserves. Nevertheless, cluttering is still an orphan in the house of speech pathology—some of the most recent and complete treatises on speech disorders omit mention of it.

Cluttering is one of the most important disorders, not only of speech, but of language and communication in general. Because cluttering has a varied symptomatology and is frequently in conjunction with other speech disorders, its neglect has contributed considerably to the haziness of theoretical formulation in speech pathology and to the unreliability of reports on therapy. One of the most important developments in speech pathology in the last few decades is the recognition by an increasing

---

* The most extensive treatment of the subject is found in Liebmann's *Vorlesungen über Sprachstörungen* (Berlin: Coblentz, 1890) and, excluding the case histories cited, the passage does not exceed twelve pages.
† R. Luchsinger, *Das Poltern* (Cluttering) (Berlin-Charlottenburg: C. Marhold, 1963).

number of therapists that cluttering has a close and intricate relationship with stuttering. Both disorders seem to belong to the same family, but stuttering, as the major speech disorder, has so completely overshadowed its "illegitimate" brother that many speech therapists are still unable to make a differential diagnosis. Indeed, clutterers often consult therapists about "stuttering" that simply does not exist.

This volume, like the others of the series, is intended primarily for practicing speech therapists and students. Accordingly we have omitted discussion of some of the more philosophical problems which might not be of immediate concern to the practitioner. The theories in this book are derived from clinical observation and from the author's long therapeutic experience in speech pathology.

We regret that the systematic research cited here is unduly meager, but this merely reflects the regrettable lack of attention accorded to cluttering. In the White House Surveys, for example, no incidence of cluttering was reported because no category bearing that name was included in the studies. Some clutterers undoubtedly found their way into the reported figures on stuttering, articulatory problems, and delayed speech.

The international literature on speech pathology is somewhat more concerned with cluttering than the American literature. We cite it when appropriate and hope that the non-English references will not be a burden to the reader.

The predominant reason for the omission of cluttering from the literature is probably the fact that the majority of clutterers do not seek professional help. Thus it is impossible even to estimate the extent of the statistical incidence of cluttering in the general population. Clutterers remain uncounted, but communicatively handicapped, and apparently more disturbing to their listeners than to themselves. Although unaware of their handicap, they need the help of therapists who are familiar with their problem.

The seemingly novel and possibly controversial concepts set forth here are actually a reassessment and rearrangement of the

elements of theory and practice which are familiar to all sea-
soned speech pathologists. We hope that it will lead to more
effective therapy and to further research. The interested student
will find many hypotheses in need of systematic validation.

We are indebted not only to the numerous authors quoted,
but also to many young colleagues whose searching questions
obliged us to clarify a number of issues. However, we have not
attempted to camouflage any gap in our knowledge. Meaningful
discovery is more apt to be made when questions remain open
rather than buried under the verbiage of inadequate answers.

I am deeply grateful to Dr. Charles Van Riper for his suggestion that a book such as this be written, and for his constant and
active interest. Some chapters are a direct offshoot of our discussions. Mrs. Leila Shapira prepared the manuscript with excep-
tional care and ability.

Acceptance of the theories expounded here may be a slow
process, but we look forward more immediately to the results of
further research and inquiry which this volume hopefully will
foster.

D.A.W.

To my dear wife

Renata

for her inspiration, dedication, and forbearance.

contents

CLUTTERING IS A SPEECH DISORDER CHARACTERIZED BY THE CLUT-
terer's unawareness of his disorder, by a short attention span,
by disturbances in perception, articulation and formulation of
speech and often by excessive speed of delivery. It is a disorder
of the thought processes preparatory to speech and based on a
hereditary disposition. Cluttering is the verbal manifestation of
Central Language Imbalance, which affects all channels of communication (e.g. reading, writing, rhythm and musicality) and
behavior in general.

1

the problem of cluttering

HISTORY

The history of cluttering begins with the anecdotes of antiquity. Battaros, a legendary Lybian king, spoke quickly and in
a disorderly fashion, and others who spoke as he did were said
to suffer from *battarismus*. Demosthenes, the greatest of the
Greek orators, was supposed to have been cured of stuttering by
Satyros, the famous actor and voice teacher (*phonaskos*). In our
opinion Demosthenes was a clutterer. Plutarch describes his
symptoms as excessive temperament, indistinct speech, some dyslalia, weak voice, short breath, and inability to focus on the
main point of discourse. In addition, the nature of the exercise
he performed suggests that cluttering was the disorder he was
trying to overcome.

1   The literature and argumentation of this much discussed question is well
     summarized in H. Holst, "Demosthenes' Speech Impediment," *Symbolae*
     Osloenses (Oslo), fasc. 4 (1926), pp. 11-25.

Even these few early references to what we know as cluttering
reflect the double historical aspect of the disorder: first, the
manifest history, in which cluttering was recognized as a distinct
disorder, and second, the covert history, in which cluttering was
confused with or subsumed under stuttering. We shall consider
the manifest history, with an occasional reference to the covert
history.

Hippocrates's *(99)* famous theory that stuttering is a result of
improper balance between thought and speech is actually more
applicable to cluttering. However, throughout antiquity and the
Middle Ages cluttering was not identified as a distinct phenomenon. In the light of our present knowledge it can be seen
that the works of Aetius (sixth century), Hieronymus Mercurialis (1584), and a few others contain faint foreshadowings of
reference to cluttering as a separate disorder, but they belong,
nonetheless, to the prehistory of cluttering.

David Bazin (1717) contributed a remarkable description and
analysis of cluttering in his book *De lingua et ejus vitiis mor-
bosis* in his chapter on stuttering as quoted in Luchsinger
(121:178-83):

> Then there is a bad habit, acquired in childhood and not cor-
> rected by the parents, a restless and too labile disposition which
> causes the tongue to outstrip the thoughts or that several un-
> necessary thoughts and ideas try to get expressed at the same time;
> making the effort to proffer them in the same instant, the speaker
> cannot keep them asunder and gets stuck in the first syllable,
> blocking with his tongue.... Here we have to mention also an
> over-hurrying of speech when these individuals, due to their
> excessive speech drive, don't take sufficient time for the correct
> enunciation of words. In such individuals speech is often quicker
> than their thoughts and they mostly try to express ideas which are
> as yet incoherent and chaotic.

Bazin also adds that this disturbance depends more upon the
mind than upon the tongue.

It was only during the beginning of the nineteenth century that cluttering was differentiated from stuttering. In 1830 Marc Colombat (de l'Isère) used the current French expressions *bredouillement* to indicate excessive rapidity leading to poor articulation and *balbutiement* to indicate hesitation resulting from inability to find the appropriate word or phrase. Dr. Serre d'Alais (1841), a clutterer himself, described his own symptoms with utmost clarity, and for therapy suggested a slower tempo and clarification of thought before speech. He considered himself a "not fully developed stutterer."

Joseph Poett, Sr. (*163*) wrote in 1833: "A very common species of impediment usually designated *stuttering*, frequently originates with children, in consequence of the impatience, excitement or rapidity of utterance, with which their nursery governess or any other persons may be habituated to whom the child is intrusted to receive the rudiments of education ... certain letters of words of one syllable are reiterated or often repeated ... and the child gradually degenerates into a complete stutterer." Poett attributed the "exciting cause" to a "debility of nervous energy" and advised "prosodial instruction." (He spoke of the disorder we designate as *cluttering*, because the spasmodic disorder of speech he called *stammering*.)

Almost a century ago, Adolf Kussmaul, the greatest lexicographer in the field of speech pathology, employed his diversified medical knowledge in preparing an astounding treatise on speech and speech disorders. [1] He states that the term *cluttering* had been used previously by English authors. Kussmaul describes the symptoms clearly, emphasizing that although the disorder can easily be confused with stuttering, the two differ in that cluttering "improves when the patient pays attention to what he is saying." Investigators of the next few decades added little to the knowledge of the disorder. They cited Kussmaul's description of cluttering, and, as he did, prescribed exercises in

---

[1] It appeared almost simultaneously with the German edition in Ziemssen, *Cyclopedia of the Practice of Medicine* (New York: William Wood, 1877), XIV, 581-875.

rhythm and concentrated attention to speech details. There was
no significant contribution between the time of Kussmaul's treatise and 1900, when Albert Liebmann (119) published a comprehensive study of the subject. Liebmann described the symptoms of cluttering more precisely than had been done previously
and introduced his finding that cluttering can result from either
motor or sensory disabilities and that therapy must differ according to the type. Subsequent writings of the next three decades
added little to Liebmann's contribution. During this period
only the German literature (92 and 148:359-480) considered
cluttering as a distinct pathological entity.

In 1916 James Sonnet Greene (87) described a case which he
called *agitophasia,* pointing out that the disorder also affected
the patient's handwriting. Berkhan (1889) had previously noted
(20) the concomitance of speech and writing disorders, and in
1926 Klara Roman-Goldzieher began her expansion of this line
of research. C. S. Bluemel, a stutterer himself, attempted to
study all of the relevant literature in order to find a cure for
stuttering. His own theory of primary stammering, which he
began to publish in 1913 (25), can be considered a direct pre-
cursor of the current theory of the interrelationship of cluttering and stammering. The second edition of Emil Froeschels'
textbook (75) on speech and voice disorders (1932) marked an
important step forward because it attempted to explore the psychological mechanism underlying cluttering. Florensky (68:159-
78) made a significant contribution in 1933 when she stated
conclusively that accelerated speech (tachylalia) is a symptom,
rather than the essence, of cluttering, and is not always manifested by the clutterer. However, at this time, despite the presence of a large number of known therapeutic measures—sum-
marized by D. A. Weiss (217:34-35) in 1936—the prognosis for
cluttering was doubtful at best.

A new era of heightened interest in cluttering began when
H. Freund and D. A. Weiss, working independently, started

gathering evidence that stuttering may have its roots in cluttering. Earlier investigators had noted that cluttering and stuttering sometimes co-exist, but Freund (70:1446-57 and Weiss (215: 1-4) defined the basic clinical relationship of the two disorders. In 1935 Koukol and Poray-Koshitz (115:171-78), disciples of Florensky, gave their enthusiastic support to the theory. (Since then cluttering seems to have practically disappeared from the Russian literature.)

Cluttering would have continued to exist on the periphery of speech pathology—principally because of the typical clutterer's failure to seek treatment—were it not for the relationship of cluttering and stammering. In 1950 Weiss (219) suggested that cluttering, a hereditary disorder with an "organic flavor," might be only one aspect of a generalized disorder of all channels of communication. He called the general disorder *Central Language Imbalance*. Many other speech pathologists accepted the validity of this concept. Publication of this theory and another by Freund (1952) on the interrelationship of stuttering and cluttering (71:146-68) inspired an increasing number of publications on both sides of the Atlantic, culminating in an extended section on cluttering in the second edition of the Luchsinger-Arnold (5:672-84) textbook (1952), in Seeman's (190) treatise on speech disorders (1959), and in the first complete volume devoted to cluttering, written by Luchsinger (126) in 1963.

At present, intensive research on cluttering is being carried out in various centers: in Zurich under the direction of Dr. Richard Luchsinger, in Prague under Professor Miloslav Seeman, and at the National Hospital for Speech Disorders in New York under Dr. Godfrey Arnold. Within the last few years an increasing number of publications on cluttering have appeared in the American literature, although some textbooks still fail even to mention it. In the interest of successful speech therapy we hope that cluttering will finally assume its rightful position in the field of speech pathology.

Many disturbances in communication, such as delayed speech, dyslalias, cluttering, stuttering, reading difficulties, and disturbances of rhythm and musicality, were thought to be unrelated entities, although their frequent coincidence was often noted. However, the complexity of the symptomatology of cluttering, together with the observation that cluttering is interrelated with other speech disorders, indicated that a more general pathological basis might underlie all of these problems. In 1950 D. A. Weiss (*221:252-62*) suggested that this common pathological basis of language and communication disorders be called *Central Language Imbalance*. The prime characteristics of Central Language Imbalance are lack of concentration, short attention span, and lack of awareness of the functions of communication; the term also indicates that the degree of severity of these characteristics varies from case to case.

Cluttering is the manifestation of Central Language Imbalance in the area of verbal utterance. The term describes the disorderly and often overaccelerated manner of speaking which is the external expression of the unclear and even chaotic internal speech of those who have Central Language Imbalance.

As shown in Fig. 1, the various speech disorders can be likened to the peaks of an iceberg, which appear from a distance to emerge from the sea independently. On closer inspection, however, one notices that each peak is part of a broad mass lying beneath the surface of the water. Similarly, the various speech disorders can be seen as manifestations of a more general underlying pathology. The concept of Central Language Imbalance, or a common pathological basis of the various disorders of communication, focuses attention on related symptoms that might otherwise be overlooked. For example, a child's parents might bring him to a speech pathologist because of "stuttering." It is not unlikely that the parents would fail to note that the child also has reading difficulties, which, of course, are related to his "stuttering." Other related manifestations that

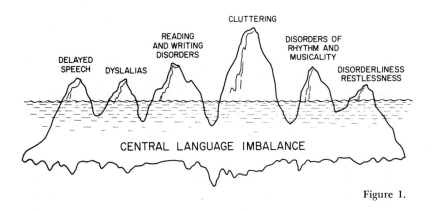

Figure 1.

the parents would be unlikely to note are lack of concentration, short attention span, untidiness, lack of musicality, lack of rhythmical sense, and so forth. The concept of Central Language Imbalance, the common denominator of many seemingly unrelated symptoms, makes it possible to ask a patient the necessary and pertinent questions.

ETIOLOGY

In typical cluttering there are no neurological symptoms, although the symptoms present have an "organic flavor." By this we mean that they run parallel to symptoms caused by an organic disease but have no concomitant neurological signs of organicity. As in organic cases, but unlike neurotic cases, concentration of attention tends to reduce cluttering symptoms and inattention aggravates them. Because cluttering symptoms are endogenous and not due to the reaction of the patient, they may be considered primary rather than secondary symptoms.

2   John Hughlings Jackson, "Speech Affections from Brain Disease," in *Selected Writings of Dr. Hughlings Jackson*, ed. J. Taylor (New York: Basic Books, 1958), pointed out in 1878 that in neurological disease, and specifically in aphasia, there are negative and positive conditions. The negative ones are the pure deficit symptoms; the positive ones indicate the reaction to the disorder. Nowadays we speak of primary symptoms,

corresponding to Jackson's deficit symptoms, and understand by
secondary ones the reaction of the patient to the awareness of his
disorder.

They constitute a basic weakness which the patient can overcome with effort—in the way that a slight limp can be cam-
ouflaged with concentrated effort, but reappears as soon as
attention slackens and effort is relaxed. The opposite is true of
stammering (stuttering), a secondary symptom, which worsens
with increased attention. The ability to improve performance
by concentrated mental effort distinguishes typical cluttering
from neurological disease with cluttering-like symptoms (see
Chapter 3). In these diseases effort hardly improves the symptoms. For purposes of comparison we can liken cluttering to an
inborn weakness, whereas neurological disease with cluttering-
like symptoms may be said to resemble almost complete paral-
ysis. In other words, the clutterer appears to be underendowed
while the organic case appears to be incapacitated.

Some authors suggest that cluttering might have a neurotic
cause.

> 3   Henry Freund (71:146-68) stresses the hereditary neurotic disposition of
>   clutterers. Scripture's (187) indications are rather terse. Compare
>   Freund's position with that of the author of the present text and also
>   with Scripture's.

However, the most constant etiological factor in cluttering
appears to be heredity. Without extensive genealogical studies,
but merely by examining the parents accompanying the patient
and eliciting information about other speech and reading disorders in the family, we generally find a history of cluttering
in the family. In order to be able to discern evidence of familial
cluttering the therapist must be thoroughly familiar with the
symptomatology. Let us cite a case in point. A well spoken
father described the cluttering symptoms of his daughter. I
asked him whether there were similar cases in the family and
he could recall none. When the patient's mother arrived later,
her painfully drawn out speech and paretic hoarseness made me
suspect that the cluttering could possibly have been inherited

from her. This seems to have been confirmed when both the mother and father agreed that the patient's maternal grand-mother spoke in a quick and "immature" manner.

The feeble-minded constitute another group in which we often find symptoms of cluttering together with a hereditary factor. Almost all the mongoloid children we have encountered manifested symptoms of cluttering. In feeble-mindedness and other cases of mental deficiency, as in organic brain disorders, cluttering is considered to be a part and consequence of the total syndrome.

4   R. Cabanas (36:34-37) tried to show that the "stuttering" of the mongoloids is, in fact, genuine cluttering.

We can conclude, then, that only when the hereditary factor is present, together with symptoms of cluttering and lack of neurological involvement, do we have a true clutterer—that is, a true case of Central Language Imbalance. When there is neurological involvement, cluttering symptoms, in our opinion, should be considered to be indicative of *symptomatic* cluttering.[2] The etiology of symptomatic cluttering is readily explainable by the neurological lesions.

There have been no pathological anatomic findings in Central Language Imbalance. The hereditary factor, therefore, raises the question of whether such a hereditary deviation should be considered organic even though no anatomical (or histological) alterations can be found. This question cannot be answered at present, but hopefully further investigation into the nature of heredity will provide the answer. The answer in turn will probably explain why particular talents or lack of talents, in varying degrees, are inherited. The clutterer, we might say, is deficient in his sense of harmony in language functions and must exert

2 The term *symptomatic* is widely used in medicine to indicate that a given symptomatology is not isolated but is part of a more generalized condition. European medical speech pathologists often designate those speech disorders which are due to neurological disorders as *symptomatic*.

effort if he wishes to speak, read, and write acceptably, just as
a musically underendowed person must exert effort if he wishes
to perform tolerably. Cluttering (Central Language Imbalance),
then, we consider to be a basic constitutional characteristic of
an individual's general disposition. The amount of the deficiency varies from case to case. However, with the correct therapeutic approach, far-reaching improvement can be achieved
in most cases.

What is the substrate of Central Language Imbalance? What
is inherited in these cases? There are a number of hypotheses,
but none can be proved or disproved at this time.

Seeman and his school (190:109-10) believe that submicro-
scopic lesions, fairly well localized in the area of the striatum,
are at the root of Central Language Imbalance. This theory
brings the problem directly into the realm of anatomy and organic lesions, placing little emphasis on the hereditary component. In light of what is known about Central Language
Imbalance, however, Katherine de Hirsch's concept (48:231-48,
49:257-61, 50:235-50, 51:3-9, 52:89-91, and 53:934-40) of lack of
maturation of the nervous system appears to be more plausible.
It does not preclude validity of the hereditary and developmental findings, and is consistent with the fact that clutterers
often appear and act younger than they are. Nonetheless, objective proof is not available, and at this time would be difficult
to obtain. Karlin (110) theorized that stuttering is caused by
delayed myelinization of the nerves, but again, there is no conclusive proof.

Falck and Falck (64:439-40) cite the lack of capacity to in-
tegrate as the most meaningful factor in what they call a *Disorder of Integrative Mechanisms*. This is certainly an important
element, but it does not account for all of the symptoms (e.g.,
lack of attention to detail). A related theory is lack of Gestalt
formation, that is, inability to organize small elements into a
meaningful whole. The element of plasticity, described in cases
of "developmental language disorders" by L. Bender (17:155-
76) may also be a consideration in cluttering. It consists of an

unsure grip on details, resulting in constantly shifting attitudes toward the same task and consequent inability to exercise control over the task at hand. Plasticity is considered a normal characteristic of young children, but when evidenced later it is a sign of lack of maturation. Present knowledge indicates that the substrate of Central Language Imbalance will be found to include some, if not all, of these elements.

The question of the substrate of Central Language Imbalance leads through various channels to the broader question of heredity of talent or lack of talent in speech and public speaking in general. It also leads to the vast area of delimitation of other disorders, such as congenital aphasia, alexia, and agraphia. The most distinctive characteristic of Central Language Imbalance, as opposed to the other disorders, is multiplicity and variety of symptoms.

Eva Sedláčková (*188*:67-77) investigated the vegetative nervous system of clutterers and stammerers. Although the final results are not yet ascertained on a sufficient number of patients, she has the impression [3] that clutterers have a certain disposition to sympathicotonia and stammerers to parasympathicotonia. Although fraught with many theoretical difficulties, this is an interesting line of investigation.

C. Guiot and his co-workers (*89*:363-80) produced acceleration of speech by electric stimulation of the region of the thalamus. R. M. Brickner (*34*:128-31) was able to produce repetition by stimulating the mesial surface of the brain in area 6 electrically. These experiments are still too few to allow any conclusion to be drawn as far as our subject is concerned, and they were undertaken on severely pathological material.

Until now we have tried to develop our theories on cluttering solely from clinical observation—from the inside out, as it were. Now we shall consider some prevailing theories in the fields of neurology and speech pathology in relation to Central Language Imbalance.

---

3 Personal communication.

The feedback principle of the activity of the Central Nervous System (C.N.S.) appears to be well founded in fact.

5   W. B. Cannon in his *Wisdom of the Body*, 2nd ed. (New York: W. W. Norton & Company, Inc., 1939) describes the self-regulation of the body which leads to homeostasis. Norbert Wiener has laid the foundations of the feedback theory; his book, *Cybernetics, or the Control and Communication in the Animal and the Machine* (New York: John Wiley & Sons, Inc., 1949) is very worthwhile to read and the omission of some pages of mathematical symbols does not interrupt the continuity.

It is based on the concept that during every controlled bodily movement proprioceptive information on the position of the moving organs is constantly fed back to the C.N.S. Awareness of the position makes control possible and it also enables us, if necessary, to correct erroneous movements during action. The feedback of the normal speaker is not very pronounced during utterance. An intelligent but phonetically untrained individual hardly knows what happens in his organs of articulation, especially in the inner cavity of the mouth, when he forms sounds. This awareness also depends upon his type of imagery. Investigators interested in phonetics report that the indigenous (savage) populations of Africa and Australia, on the other hand, can indicate more precisely on request the position of their tongue, mouth, pharynx, etc. during articulation than can the civilized population. The savage's predominantly motoric disposition possibly bears on his awareness of articulatory details. The clutterer's articulatory feedback is even less pronounced than the normal's. The clutterer, as a rule, is completely unaware of his errors and is unable to recall what he has said only a few moments previously. He is an inattentive listener and reader, and even less attentive to his own manner of speaking. Hence he finds it difficult and tiring to concentrate on correcting his speech, and can succeed for only a short time unless he is continually reminded.

Meyer-Eppler and Luchsinger (*140*:87-99), brought our attention to the role of the auditory feedback mechanism in cluttering by demonstrating that the speech disorder resulting from a delayed side tone (Lee effect) resembles cluttering rather than stuttering. As in Lee's original description (*117*:639-40 and *118*:824-26), only symptoms of disorganized speech were noticed, without the characteristic spasmodic blocks of stammering. Following a lead supplied by Wolf and Wolf (*230*:48-61), Arnold (*9*:14-23) has recently suggested that cluttering be viewed in the light of a delay in the auditory feedback which results from sensory dysgnosia (difficulty in perceiving sensory impressions).[4] Taking into account the lag in motor feedback which derives from the "syndrome of congenital dyspraxia," Arnold considers cluttering in the light of deficient homeostasis. (Homeostasis can be maintained only by a well functioning feedback system.) Probably more appropriate would be a term which would parallel *homeostasis* (maintenance of equilibrium) but denotes in addition the concept of well balanced functioning. No such term is as yet available. The study and testing of theories such as these, growing out of the application of theoretical material in related fields, hopefully will lead to new discoveries relevant to Central Language Imbalance and keep our theories abreast of current thought.

Communication theory illuminates some basic characteristics of cluttering. In the interpersonal communication circuit,

6   Communication theory and cluttering have been discussed by G. Arnold
    (9:14-23). Communication theory is aptly—but too mathematically—summarized by J. R. Pierce, *Symbols, Signals and Noise* (New York: Harper
    & Row, Publishers, 1961). A good general introduction is provided
    by G. A. Miller, *Language and Communication* (New York-Toronto-London: McGraw-Hill Book Company, 1951), and the more clinical and
    psychiatric aspects are treated in J. Ruesch, "General Theory of Communication in Psychiatry," in the *American Handbook of Psychiatry*, ed.
    S. Arieti (New York: Basic Books, 1959), I, 895-908.

the clutterer's relationship with his interlocutor appears to be more superficial than that of the normal speaker. In addition to being a poor listener, the clutterer does not seem to be con-

4 This point of view calls to mind Hoepfner's (*100*:16-57) conception of stammering. Without the knowledge that cluttering is the basis of stammering, Hoepfner considered stammering to be a kind of sensory aphasia.

cerned with expressing himself comprehensibly. His interest is
more in unburdening himself rather than in communicating.
His nonverbal communication—that is, his gestures and facial
movements—is more lively than that of the average speaker,
but his intonation is more stereotyped and monotonous. Clut-

> 7   L. Kaiser (107:95-104) proposes the expressions *nonverbal, preverbal,*
> *primitive,* or *biological* for this part of human expression. Compare these
> concepts with those of J. Hughlings Jackson (see Search Item No. 2) on
> emotional language.

terers, then, are poor communicators. Until now no systematic
attempt has been made to describe cluttering from the frame
of reference of communication theory.

Godfrey Arnold (6:25-45) dealt with the question of left-
handedness and changing of handedness in cluttering. He considers the whole problem very nebulous and does not attribute
any specific importance to it as far as our subject is concerned.
We feel inclined to agree with him. Shifting handedness and
similar problems might exert some unspecific pressure on the
child, possibly aggravating already existing difficulties, but not
creating them originally.

The ability to speak progresses from the infant's initial stage
of globality by differentiation into progressively more refined
details. Froeschels [5] has recently stressed the importance of this
fact in relation to stammering. During his speech blocks the
stammerer completely loses the global aspect of speech and
focuses pathologically exaggerated attention on small details of
his verbal delivery. In cluttering, on the other hand, we have
the impression that globality remains in the foreground, dis-
arranging and distorting many details which are necessary for
an orderly and integrated delivery and often even for compre-
hensibility. In this respect cluttering resembles infantile speech.
This observation leads us back to the most plausible explanation of the substrate of Central Language Imbalance, namely,
unevenness and lag in maturation.

> [5] "Structure of Speech and Stuttering." Lecture at the *New York*
> *Society for Speech and Voice Therapy,* January 9, 1963.

NOMENCLATURE

Cluttering

Cluttering has been "discovered" many times, and various authors have applied their own names to the disorder. First came the anecdotal names, such as *Battarism, Wherryism,* and *Spoonerism* (speech like that of the legendary Lybian King Battaros, Archdeacon Wherry, and Bishop Spooner). Some authors used more descriptive or scientific-sounding Latin terms, such as *tumultus sermonis* (chaotic speech), *agitophasia* (excited speech), *tachyphemia* (quick speech), and *paraphrasia praeceps* (speech formulation distorted by overhurrying).

> 8   M. Ogilvie (152) summarized in 1942 the international research on clut-
> tering and collected twenty-three synonyms in the English literature. Her
> work is remarkable for its time.

The English word *cluttering* hints at the basic disorderliness of the disturbance. The German *Poltern* denotes a disorderly noise, and the North German *Bruddeln* suggests a precipitated spouting of noises. The Hungarian *hadarás* is indicative of over-hurried speech with resulting indistinctness. The Spanish *tartajeo* means general precipitous disorderliness, and to replace this commonly used word I suggested *tartaleo,* which has a similar connotation but is not in common usage. The Italian *tartagliare,* like the Spanish term, is probably onomatopoetic and denotes repetitiousness.[6] Recently the word *abburattamento,* meaning disorderliness, has been applied. The various symptoms of cluttering are differentiated more finely in French than in other languages. *Bredouillement* is used commonly to mean embarrassed and overhurried speech; *balbutiement* means hesitation and repetition caused by inability to find the necessary words in time; *bâfouillement* means talking in circles without being able to come to the point; and *ânonnement* means the

---

6 Bilancioni (21) quotes an anecdote which purports that the word originated with the sixteenth-century musician Tartaglia, whose speech was supposedly marked by repetition.

interjection of vowels (*ah-ah-ah*) by speakers who cannot find
the next word. In German this interjection of vowels is called
Gaxen (*Staxen*), a rarely used word. The list of labels could go
on interminably, but we have cited enough to indicate that the
public has generally been quicker than the professionals to
recognize and name the speech disorder that we know as cluttering.

9   Does the existence in so many languages of a term for cluttering indicate
    its validity as a disorder? See Wendell Johnson, "The Indians Have No
    Word for It," *Quarterly Journal of Speech*, XXX (1944), 330-37 and
    456-65.

The word *cluttering* was definitely known among British
speech pathologists by the second half of the nineteenth century.
The origin of the expressive term unfortunately is not known.
It apparently is related to *clatter, cluster,* and *clot.* We may hope
that the word will be used more frequently in the American
literature, where it has rarely been recognized as a distinct disorder, even though its symptomatology has been discussed.

Stuttering and Stammering

James Hunt (*103*), quoting Adelung (1786), says that *stuttering* refers to repetitions and *stammering* to spasmodic blocks in
speech. Most of the British and some of the early American authors followed this rule, although there were numerous excep-
tions. (One of them was Hunt himself.) In recent years the two
expressions have come to be regarded as basically synonymous,
especially in the American literature and the term *stammering*
acquired some disrepute through the frequent use by quack
experts who promised to cure all stammerers quickly in their
stammering schools.

Because of the important confusions and connections between
cluttering and stuttering we have had to consider here the use
of the alternate term, stammering. The word *stuttering* unfortunately has become rather imprecise and generalized. In pop-
ular usage it seems to include stammering, cluttering, and also

at times those mistakes of disfluency that people make because of momentary embarrassment or uncertainty. Thus the vague term *stuttering* often denotes a disorder more like cluttering than does the specific term *stammering*. If someone is called a *stutterer*, we do not know whether he is a clutterer, an unsure

10   The problem of defining stuttering has been an important one and is far from being solved. See C. S. Bluemel, "Concepts of Stammering; A Century in Review," *Journal of Speech and Hearing Disorders*, XXV (1960), 24-32.

and hesitant speaker, or whether he is suffering from the major speech disorder characterized by spasmodic blocking and fear of speech. When we say he is a *stammerer*, we mean only this last category.

We mildly regret this deviation from the usual terminology, though it appears to us to be both logical and convenient. It makes our differential diagnosis more precise. We trust that the term *stammering* to represent the spasmodic and fearful speech disorder often called *secondary stuttering* will present no semantic difficulties to the reader of this text. We need it to make our position clear.

11   The vagueness of the term stuttering has bothered many speech pathologists. A critical review of the divergent opinions can be found in P. J. Glasner and F. D. Vermilyea, "An investigation of the Definition and Use of the Diagnosis 'Primary Stuttering,' " *Journal of Speech and Hearing Disorders*, XVIII (1953), 161-67.

Central Language Imbalance

In 1950 we published our theory of a common (and hereditary) pathology underlying various language disorders. Cluttering is the manifestation of this pathology in the area of speech delivery. We called this common pathology *Central Language Imbalance*. Several speech pathologists have since suggested other names: Luchsinger, asthenia (weakness) of speech (*122:7-14*), and Arnold, General Language Disability (*6:25-45*). Falck and Falck (*64:439-40*), unaware of publication of our theory, hypothesized the existence of this common element, calling it *Disturbance of Nervous Integration* (DNI).* Each of these terms suggests one or another aspect, but not the entire concept of what we call Central Language Imbalance. Leaving the defense of their nomenclature to the respective authors, we shall explain our own preference for the term *Central Language Imbalance*.

The disorder is *central* in the sense of bearing on numerous functions and also in originating in the brain. *Language* connotes all channels of communication, and Central Language Imbalance can affect all functions of communication. *Imbalance* is not commonly used in this sense, and thus we can endow it with a specific meaning, which is advantageous in the case of a new concept. It suggests, on the one hand, lack of harmony in the functioning of various elements, but does not suggest a specific cause. Indeed, the cause is unknown. On the other hand, it hints at the possibility that equilibrium can be re-established by re-inforcing the elements which do not "pull their weight." It also indicates that the new balance can be maintained only if effort is exerted continuously to compensate for the innate instability. If an exact and specific cause for Central Language Imbalance is found, a more appropriate label can be applied accordingly. ᠅᠅᠅

* Worth mentioning are the expressions Minimal Brain Damage (in W. C. Barger, "Neuropsychiatric Diagnosis in Minimal Brain Damage," *Proceedings of the Rip Van Winkle Clinic*, II (1960), 13-25) and Infantile Speech and Language Organization Impairments (in J. B. de Quirós, "Dysphasia and Dyslexia in School Children," *Folia Phoniatrica*, XVI (1964), 201-22). They refer to the possibility of a common basis of speech and reading disorders, also suspected by several authors quoted in the bibliography.

REPETITION OF ONE-SYLLABLE WORDS OR THE FIRST SYLLABLE OF polysyllabic words is an imporant symptom of cluttering. These repetitions may occur occasionally in normal speech also; most frequently when the speaker is under pressure. In both cluttering and normal speech it is a sign that the speaker is uncertain of the word or phrase to follow. The "speech motors are idling" while the business of speaking continues without being fueled by words.

Repetition of syllables is common and normal in children, especially between the ages of two and five, when the substance

symptoms

of what the child wishes to communicate is too complex for expression in his limited vocabulary. During these years the

> 12   Two publications, *Stuttering in Children and Adults* (Minneapolis, Minn.: University of Minnesota Press, 1955) and *The Onset of Stuttering* (Minneapolis, Minn.: University of Minnesota Press, 1959), both edited by Wendell Johnson *et al.*, should be read in context with the article by M. E. Wingate, "Evaluation and Stuttering, Part I. Speech Characteristics of Young Children," *Journal of Speech and Hearing Disorders,* XXVII (1962), 106-15, for a comprehensive review of the literature on normal repetition in children.

inception of cluttering, if it is uncomplicated by stammering [1] or other disorders, may be overlooked. Diagnosis cannot be

> [1] *Stammering* is used in this text to denote the disorder characterized by spasmodic blocks, and *stuttering* is by-passed as a popular catch-all by various unspecified speech disorders. As we have explained in the chapter on nomenclature, we have special reasons for this usage.

confirmed until other symptoms, such as excessive speed and disorderliness, become apparent.

The rate of speed of a clutterer's repetition is the exact syllabic speed of his nonrepetitive (or free-flowing) speech. This is true also of the repetition of normals under stress and is an important factor in differential diagnosis. A faster or slower rate indicates that the individual has become aware of his repeating and is attempting to correct it: corrective awareness of disorder rules out cluttering as we define it. The clutterer's characteristic unawareness of his speech deviation accounts for his continuing to make syllabic noises (repetition of syllables) instead of stopping the speech process while he decides on the words to follow. Children whose repetition is characteristic of a phase of speech development are also unaware of the fact that they repeat. When a child becomes aware of his repetition and tries to correct it, the rate becomes slower as Froeschels (75) has made clear.

In most cases of stammering there is repetition at the same rate as nonrepetitive speech in the early phases. This indicates a cluttering component (cluttering-stammering). Repetition at a faster or slower rate than free-flowing speech indicates conscious attempt at correction and hence the danger of development of stammering.

Excessive speed (tachylalia)

Until recently excessive speed was considered the most significant symptom of cluttering, and some investigators even considered it the basic element. However, there are some normals who speak too rapidly but with perfect order and articulation and there are clutterers who speak at a normal rate. Therefore excessive speed must be ruled out as the one prime indicator of cluttering. An abnormally fast delivery may annoy or frustrate a listener, but we tend to consider it normal nonetheless when it is a comfortable rate for the speaker and is unaccompanied by other symptoms, such as hesitation or repetition. For example, there are professors whose formulations are brilliant and whose delivery is flawless; but, the rate of their delivery is too fast for effortless reception by students. In these cases high speed seems to be an indicator that the speech mechanism is able to cope with the larger-than-normal burden imposed by a higher-than-average intelligence and a strong drive to communicate.

In cluttering, on the other hand, when there is excessive speed it is accompanied by poor formulation and delivery, and is therefore an indicator that the speech mechanism cannot cope with its function of communication.

A clutterer will sometimes begin polysyllabic words at an acceptable rate, but his speed increases as he progresses, resulting in a "telescoping" of the word. He apparently has a global impression of a word and hence pronounces it in a single spurt. He spells as he pronounces, omitting the same letters. This also occurs in some speech disorders that are a result of brain lesions (e.g., postencephalitic speech). Seeman (*191*:170-76) called it *interverbal acceleration*. Luchsinger (*125*:804-13) added the concept of *intraverbal acceleration* in cluttering. The first indicates the shortening or omission of the essential pauses between words (where a comma or period is indicated in written matter). Cognizance of these would-be punctuation marks is a requirement of good speaking. D. Bradford (*33*:59-65) says correctly that "silence is just as much a part of speech as articulation." Intraverbal acceleration leads to the contraction of longer words.

Almost every writer on cluttering notes the powerful drive behind all the clutterer's activities. However, as in his speech, his general performance is poor, or at best uneven. The excessive speed with which most—but not all—clutterers speak characterizes all their undertakings. Gerstmann and Schilder (*84*:570-86) and Seeman (*190*) attempted to localize the anatomical site of this speed drive and concluded that it is in the striopallidar system of the brain. Ungovernable speed is seen with lesions of this system, especially in encephalitis, but there are no available histological findings at this time for clutterers. Given the hereditary factor in typical cluttering, however (see page 52), it is not anticipated that structural changes in the brain will be found to cause the excessive speed.

Discussion of the role of another process is relevant here. Normal conscious action is constantly controlled by the feedback mechanism. That is, the brain constantly receives tactile, visual, and auditory information, and signals indicating the movements or position of the limbs or other structures. The clutterer's feedback mechanism seems to provide less-than-normal conscious control. If a typical clutterer, for instance, reads a short text or performs a simple task, only a few minutes later he might be unable to recall the content of what he has read or the nature of what he has done. Future research may determine the role of this lack of control as a factor in excessive speed.

Unfortunately, determination of the normal rate of speed presents considerable difficulties. When the calculation is made, several factors will have to be considered. First, people in southern countries generally speak at a faster rate than those in northern countries. Mexican Spanish, for instance, is slow and drawn out compared to the whirlwind speed of Cuban Spanish. The drawl of the southern United States is an exception to this rule. Second, the rural population generally speaks at a slower rate than the urban population. Normal speed, then, must be determined regionally. In addition, age, habit, and the emotional importance of what is being said influence the speed of speech. Calculation of the limits of "normal" speed, with these factors accounted for, would be a valuable study.

13   The normal rate of good American speech was given as 140-180 words per minute by Hanley and Thurman (97). There are, however, great variations of rate, depending upon the emotions involved, say Kelly and Steer (111:222-26). They also discuss the principles which should orient future research in this field. Hanley and Thurman (97) also discuss the effect of the rate of utterance upon intelligibility and the pause duration effects. The positive influence on the emphasis by reducing the rate of speech was investigated by Tiffin and Steer (203).

Dumke and his associates (57:155-69) compared clutterers' spontaneous rate of speed with their speed when speaking "carefully" and found the spontaneous rate higher in each case (by as much as 300 per cent in some cases). Many clutterers do not speak with excessive speed when compared to the average population. Froeschels (77:31-33) writes that these clutterers probably speak "relatively too quickly," that is, at a rate too fast for their own ability to find words and formulate sentences. Some clutterers speak rather slowly, but nevertheless draw out the final syllables of words or interject elongated vowels (*ah-ah-ah* or *a-a-a*) in an attempt to maintain the speed and continuity of long exposition.

H. H. Beebe (15:273-76) asked sixty normal subjects to talk and to read as fast as possible, and compared their delivery with their usual manner of speaking. During this "voluntary tachylalia" symptoms of cluttering appeared in most of the subjects, even in those who were not able to increase their rate of speed. This proves that tachylalia—or even the suggestion of haste—can produce cluttering symptoms. On the other hand, if no such symptoms appear in a fast speaker, we cannot speak of cluttering.

In summary we can state that clutterers speak too quickly relative to their own ability, but not necessarily when compared to the average population. Diagnosis of cluttering cannot be made on the basis of the speed of speech alone. An individual can be diagnosed a clutterer only when his speech shows signs of faulty integration.

DRAWLING AND INTERJECTIONS

The clutterer's inability to find the words he needs in sufficient time to maintain a smooth flow of speech causes him to prolong vowels, most often at the ends of words (67:1241-44). This is in effect a stalling device during which he searches for the next word. Occasionally a clutterer will prolong a vowel at the beginning of a word, in which case it would appear that the cause of prolongation cannot be the quest for the same word. On questioning clutterers, however, we find that when they prolong a vowel at the beginning of a word, they are in the process of searching for the next word before completing verbalization of the word they have begun. This is consistent with the clutterer's overacceleration of speech and disharmony of reading and verbalization rates when reading aloud. He reads much faster than he verbalizes. One of our clutterers complained that he often seemed to be "ahead of himself."

The frantic quest for the next word also causes clutterers to interject single vowels such as *ah,* consonants such as *mm,* articulatory combinations such as *ahem,* and words such as *well* and *you know* more often than normal speakers. As the clutterer becomes more relaxed in a given situation his use of interjections increases. Normal speakers and stammerers, on the other hand, use interjections more frequently when under tension or when a situation demands a careful choice of words.

A clutterer sometimes prolongs the interjections (*ah* - - - - or *mm* - - - -), and remains unaware of their presence in his speech, although his listeners find them utterly tiresome. As we have noted earlier, the Germans call these prolonged interjections *Gaxen* or *Staxen;* the French liken them to the braying of a donkey: *âner* or *ânonner.*

Because the clutterer is inept at finding the necessary words to express his ideas, his speech is studded with clichés and repetition of words and phrases. A normal speaker has more ability in varying his means of expression.

VOWEL STOP

Vowel stop consists of a stop before pronunciation of the initial vowel, with the mouth open as if frightened.[2] Early therapists considered vowel stop appearing in conjunction with unimpaired ability to pronounce the initial consonant to be one of the important symptoms of cluttering. Liebmann *(119)* considers it a decisive symptom in the differential diagnosis. It

---

[2] The incidence of vowel stop seems higher among (Northern) German clutterers, although it is found occasionally in other clutterers. This is probably because the Northern German idiom permits and even encourages a glottal stop on the initial vowel.

is especially common at the beginning of a new phrase or sentence.

Blocking on the initial vowel exists among stammerers, but it is not a common occurrence. Pure vowel stammerers are extremely rare. The essential difference between the stammerer's *spasmodic* blocking and the clutterer's simple vowel stop is the fact that the clutterer is unaware of his hesitation and consequently does not develop a fearful attitude toward the sound. The stammerer stops as a result of a phobic reaction to a particular sound, whereas the clutterer stops as a result of his inability to find the next word in sufficient time. When he finds the necessary word, the clutterer rushes on his heedless way. Vowel stop is particularly common among mentally retarded clutterers and is particularly characteristic of the speech of mongoloids (36:34-37).

Articulation and motor disabilities

Every investigator in the field has noted the clutterer's poor articulation. It is characterized by superficiality and lack of precision, even when the pacing of syllables is correct. Blandness and lack of expressiveness characterize pronunciation—paralleling, we might say, the monotony of delivery.

Inexpressive articulation (as well as lack of inflection or stereotyped intensity and pitch patterns) is more pronounced when speech is too rapid. It is for this reason too that clutterers are frequently incapable of being understood. Many clutterers come for consultation with the complaint: "People say that they cannot understand me and I don't know why." As treatment progresses they often report that they are asked less frequently to repeat.

Albert Liebmann (*119*) specifies these deviations: (*a*) omission of sounds, syllables, and whole words (ellipsis), (*b*) displacement of sounds (heterotopy), (*c*) inversion of the order of sounds (metathesis), (*d*) anticipation of sounds, (*e*) postposition of sounds; and (*f*) repetition of initial sounds. We would add another item, i.e., *(g)* telescoping of several syllables of a word. Liebmann says that these deviations improve when speed is reduced, whereas articulation in normal speech does not change as a function of speed.

Because of the clutterer's lack of distinct articulation and rapid delivery, it is difficult to describe, or more aptly to transcribe, his articulatory deviations. Shepherd *(194*:73-81) provides us with some transcriptions of cluttered speech in the international phonetic alphabet. Figure 2 is an example of the description of a trip to the hospital by a fourteen-year-old clutterer of

A

Well,   I took the Palm Bay   train to 125th Street

wɛl | aɪ tʊk ðə ʹpɑm ʹbeɪ | ʌ | ʹtreɪn tʊəʹhʌnʹtwɛɪʹfiθ ʹstrit

and got off and changed to the express

| ən ʹgɑt ʹɔf æn ʹtʃeɪndʒ tə ʹdjɛkʹsprɛs

to 14th Street   and I walked   I think five blocks

tʊ ʹfɔʹtinθ strit | naɪ ʹwɔkt | θɪŋk ʹfaɪv. ʹblɑks | |

I think it is   five.

aɪ ʹθiŋk ɪt ɪz | | faɪv | |

B

No, I get dizzy when I read on subway trains.

noʊ | aɪjaɪgɛdɪzɪəjaɪʹrɪdɑ̃ ʹsʌbweɪ ʹtreɪnz | |

Figure. 2. Phonetic analysis of the speech of a fourteen-year-old clutterer of better-than-average intelligence *(A)*. After several months of therapy the patient has acceptable speech, but still clutters in excited moments *(B)*. After Shepherd *(194:*73-81).

better-than-average intelligence. In Figure 3 a seventeen-year-old clutterer answers questions about his studies and about his family.

My aunt   came over   to   my house,   and I played
maɪ 'ænt | | kəm'oʊvə | tu | | mʌ'haʊs | æn aɪ'pleɪd

basketball.   I was playing   basketball   by
'bæskəbɔl | | aɪ wəz 'pleɪn | | 'bæskəbɔl | | ʌm 'baɪ |

my house   on   University Avenue.
mʌ'haʊs | | ɑn | jʊnɪ'vɜsɪtɪæ̃vənjʊ | |

Well, I'm taking Physics.   That's giving me a little
wɛlə'teɪkən 'fiziks | ðæts givə mɪ ə 'lɪdəl

trouble.   I don't do as well as I did in Biology
'trʌbəl | aɪ doʊʔ dʊ əz wɛl əz ʌ dɪdən 'baɪ'ɑlədʒɪ |

and General Science.   Well, there are some
'dʒɛnrəl 'saɪənts | | wɛl ðɛr səm

complicated formulas you have to memorize.
'kɑmpləkeɪtəd 'fɔrmjələż jəhæftə'mɛmraɪz |

That's mainly the problem, I guess.
'smeɪnlɪ ðə 'prɑbləm aɪ gɛs | |

Well,   I have one brother. I have a mother and a
wɛl | a hæv'wʌn 'brʌðɚ əhævə'mʌðɚnə

father.   They're both living.
'faðə | ə 'boʊθ 'lɪvɪŋ | |

Figure. 3. A seventeen-year-old clutterer answers questions about his studies and about his family. After G. Shepherd (*194*:73-81).

Such a transcription fails to reflect the vagueness and confusion of the clutterer's articulation. The listener is often hard
put to choose the most similar conventional sound. Shepherd
remarks pertinently: "There is a constant error running through
all [these transcriptions]. The phonetic text makes the speech
look intelligible. *Some* of it was in fact intelligible; otherwise
no transcription would have been feasible; but at many points,
it was necessary to replay the tape twenty or more times in
order to determine (1) *what* was said and (2) h*ow* it was said
in [phonetic terms]. What the symbols cannot represent is the
whirlwind speed of utterance."

Nonetheless, in these short transcriptions we can notice some
embolophrasies (interjections). Such interjected syllables have
the same role as *well, huh, look,* etc. They are stallers rather
than starters. As in the case of repetitions they serve to allow
time for the clutterer to seek the next word. The most common
of these interjections is "you know. . . ." When we respond with
"you say 'you know' because you don't know," we get an embarrassed admission that this is true.

Clearer and often more humorous are the syllabic confusions
such as the famous Sperryism: "The Lord is a shoving leopard"
(loving shepherd), and Spoonerism: "Many thinkle peep so,
I believe."

The peak of unintelligibility is reached when the syllables
fuse into one another, as though telescoping. *Parliamentarian*
becomes *pamerian, international* is changed to *inteshonal,* etc.

14   Investigate "Slurvian" in J. W. Black and W. E. Moore, *Space, Code,*
      Meaning and Communication (New York: McGraw-Hill Book Company,
      1956), IV.

On the whole the clutterer seems to exhibit his thought rather
than to communicate it. That is, he considers not the listener,
but only his own verbal discharge of a pressuring thought or
feeling. Hence he is often a terrible scourge in company, talking
incessantly and often unintelligibly.

Arnold (7:82-95) and de Hirsch (51:3-9) both noted that the

clutterer's poor articulation is paralleled by poor motor performance in general, suggesting dyspraxia (disturbance of motor
integration). Seeman and Novák (*191*:170-76) tested the articulatory ability of fifty-two clutterers and fifty-two individuals
whose speech was normal. Age, sex, and intelligence were held
constant. The test consisted of quick repetition of the syllables
pah and *tah*. The performances of the youngest subjects (ages
seven to eleven) in each group did not differ. However, clutterers over age eleven performed better than normals over age
eleven. The investigators concluded, therefore, that poor motor
skill is not the cause of poor articulation in cluttering, a conclusion which seems a bit too comprehensive for the simple
experimental design.

If clutterers have a basic motor disability, it would be reasonable to assume that performance in a given task would not
change considerably simply by drawing attention to their dys-
function. However, a clutterer's motor performance will improve considerably when it is suggested that he concentrate on
the task at hand. Therefore, evaluation of a clutterer's motor
ability should not be made on the basis of spontaneous performance, but only after he has performed a task with full
concentration.

Some clutterers manifest poor articulation with adequate motor function, and since neurological investigation reveals no
consistent deviation from the normal average, we must hypoth-
esize that poor motor performance as well as poor articulation
are the result, at least in part, of the clutterer's inadequate attention to his performance in general.

RESPIRATION

The clutterer's jerky respiration and short respiratory span
are noteworthy. Arnold (7:82-95) writes that "respiratory dysrhythmia is the first cause for the clutterer's jerky and explosive
speech." We encounter a similar problem in many areas of
speech and voice disorder and should consider it seriously in

light of possible important therapeutic implications. In some cases of primary respiratory disorder, systematic respiratory exercises are imperative.

We can label respiratory disorders *primary* if the patient manifests them not only when speaking or singing, but also in activities unrelated to phonation, as we note in cerebral palsied children. If the respiratory dysrhythmia and/or polypnea (excessive frequency of respiration and shortness of breath) are manifested only during phonation, we must assume that they are *secondary* to a speech or voice disorder.

The clutterer most often thinks and speaks in short phrases which fill the same function for him as full sentences do for the normal speaker. Froeschels (75) notes that before we speak we automatically inhale an amount of air sufficient for the length of the sentence or phrase that we intend to pronounce. Clutterers attempt only short phrases and hence must inhale more frequently. They often find themselves in an embarrassing situation because of inability to find the appropriate word, loss of the trend of their thought, and the like. Jerkiness of delivery is the cause—not the result—of their uneven respiration. This point seems to be proved when we have succeeded in slowing the clutterer's delivery and inducing him to speak in longer sentences, because we then notice neither dysrhythmia nor polypnea in his respiration.

These considerations should provide an answer to the question of whether or not we recommend respiratory exercises for clutterers. As far as we can determine, they do not influence the cluttering *per se,* but occasionally they may exert a general calming effect. Respiratory exercises fall into the category of nonspecific measures that may form a favorable foundation for the specific therapy for cluttering.

MONOTONY

Many therapists have commented on the monotony and uniformity of the clutterer's speech-melody pattern. Scripture (*187*) was the original investigator of the cause of this monotony, first

in epileptics and then in stammerers. (He did not especially
mention cluttering.) He concluded that monotony of speech
melody is related primarily to lack of musical sense, and Arnold
(*7*:82-95), Pearson (*156*:51-59), and Roman-Goldzieher (*176*:116-
39) concurred.

Although many clutterers are musically adept, nonetheless
their speech often seems to be unusually monotonous. Analysis
of the clutterer's speech melody and examination of his speech
curves by Arnold (*5*:672-84) and by Luchsinger and Dubois
(*128*:21-41) indicate that in fact he does not lack variability in
pitch. There is a short melodic pattern confined to a range
of only several notes of the scale. This pattern is repeated continually. The clutterer's speech, therefore, is not characterized
by monotony in the strict sense of the word (one tone), but by
continual repetition of a short melodic pattern. It is stereotypy
but not monotony in the sense of unchanging pitch.

Since lack of musicality does not account for lack of melodic
variation in all clutterers, D. A. Weiss (*223*:216-23) investigated
the possibility of a psychological basis for this monotony. He
found that clutterers' thoughts progressively proceed by clusters
of two or three words at a time, whereas the thoughts of normal
speakers apparently proceed by whole phrases or sentences.
Speech melody is adapted to the phrase or sentence about to
be verbalized, with projection of broader melodies for longer
phrases. Because clutterers proceed by only two or three words,
they accordingly project repeated short melodic patterns.

In therapy, as the patient learns to think a sentence through
before verbalizing it, his speech melody becomes less monotonous. At first the melody may sound artificial, but it becomes
more lifelike as the planning process becomes more natural. It
is not necessary for the therapist to bring the patient's attention
specifically to the monotony of the melody, since it can be
rectified solely as a result of planning the sentence before
verbalizing it.

15   C. S. Bluemel (28) emphasized the need to organize utterance (in stam-
      mering) and so did J. M. Fletcher, *The Problem of Stuttering* (New York:
      Longmans, Green & Co., Inc., 1928).

LACK OF RHYTHM AND MUSICAL ABILITY

Lack of rhythm in speech is one of the most readily notice-able symptoms of cluttering. [Colombat (*43*), Serre (*192*:109-10), Pearson (*156*:51-59), and others considered it the very basis of cluttering.] The majority of clutterers we have known seem to have difficulty both in perceiving and reproducing rhythmic beats. However, there are clutterers with an excellent sense of rhythm and dysrhythmic speech.

L. Pearson (*156*:51-59) administered the Drake Test for rhyth-mic ability and musical memory and the Seashore Test for recognition of rhythmic patterns to thirty-six clutterers. The results indicated that expressive dysrhythmia (inability to re-produce rhythmic patterns) is more marked than receptive dysrhythmia (inability to recognize rhythmic patterns). She suggested that clutterers perform exercises in rhythm, reason-ing that improvement in rhythmic sense would favorably affect the rhythm of speech.

G. Arnold (*9*:14-23) believes that dysrhythmia is only a part of what he calls the clutterer's *congenital amusia*. Poor pitch and poor sense of melody are often found with cluttering, but on the contrary, some clutterers have a good sense of the musi-cal elements, as the case histories of Dumke and his co-workers (*57*:155-69) and Luchsinger (*126*) reveal. Therefore, amusia can-not be considered a constitutive characteristic.

There are two categories of symptoms in cluttering: (*a*) symp-toms which are always manifested and on which diagnosis is made (obligatory symptoms) and (*b*) symptoms which are some-times manifested (facultative symptoms). There may be impair-ment of a facultative function with excellent performance of a closely related facultative function. For example, Pearson (*156*:-51-59) noted a group of child clutterers with an excellent sense of rhythm who did poorly in the other elements of musicality.

16   For the examination of rhythmical and musical ability the manuals of
       C. E. Seashore, D. Lewis, and J. G. Saetveit, *Manual of Instructions for
       the Seashore Measures of Musical Talent* (New York: Psychological Cor-

poration, 1956) and R. M. Drake, *Manual for the Drake Musical Aptitude Tests*, 2nd ed. (Chicago: Science Research Associates, 1957) are a good starting point.

CONCENTRATION AND ATTENTION SPAN

Poor concentration and short attention span are the basic symptomatic elements of cluttering. Hermann Gutzmann, Sr. *(91)* came to this conclusion as early as 1893. Attention span appears to be a function of concentration (they can be likened to the two sides of a coin), and together they constitute the basis

17   Attention span and concentration are "ill-defined concepts." D. Rapaport, *Diagnostic Psychological Testing*, 3rd printing (Chicago: The Year Book Publishers, 1945), I, 167-69, gives good working definitions.

of other symptoms of cluttering, such as reading and writing disorders. The clutterer's poor concentration precludes the ability to focus on the details of an event or an object. He approaches objects, events, and even his own activities superficially and without concentration, and therefore his memory of them is severely limited. Thus many clutterers are underachievers in school. On the other hand, if a clutterer purposefully exerts a strong effort to concentrate, he seems able to focus on detail and to remember it. He tires quickly, however, and thus the goal of therapy is to strengthen concentration and lengthen the attention span as the means of improving his communicative processes. In our experience academic performance of our clutterers improves in conjunction with successful therapy.

Attention span in verbal performance can be measured by ascertaining how many of a series of meaningless syllables a patient is able to repeat correctly after the examiner has pronounced them. In 1930 we applied this test for the first time

18   Various intelligence tests, like L. M. Terman and M. A. Merrill, *Measuring Intelligence* (Stanford-Binet) Boston: Houghton Mifflin Company, 1937), and D. Wechsler, *The Measurement of Adult Intelligence*, 3rd ed. (Baltimore: The Williams and Wilkins Company), use numeral digits for determining attention span. Metraux's article, "Auditory Memory Span for Speech Sounds," *Journal of Speech Disorders*, VII (1943), 31-38, provides other norms.

(*215*:1-4) comparing the proficiency of children with normal speech and child clutterers. Most normals could repeat three syllables at age three, four syllables at age four, and so on, until age six. From age six until puberty they could repeat one additional syllable for every two years. Other investigators cite similar or slightly less proficiency for normals, and all concur that child clutterers are less proficient than normals. Beebe (*15*:273-76) and Weiss (*217*:34-35) suggest that the attention span might best be lengthened by practice in memorizing series of meaningless syllables after hearing them pronounced once.

A practical method for detecting lapses of attention is to have the patient reduce the number 100 by 2's or 3's. This task requires constant attention, and even intelligent and mathematically adept clutterers make a surprising number of errors at first. Exercises such as this one, which demand continuous attention, are an integral part of the therapeutic program.

POORLY INTEGRATED THOUGHT PROCESSES

In the fourth century B.C. Hippocrates (*99*) noted that stutterers "think faster than they can speak." Incongruity in the speed of thought and speech is one of the first symptoms of speech disorder to be mentioned in the literature, and it is noted throughout the literature on cluttering. Clutterers or their families often cite this incongruity in a description of their problem. We must evaluate the theory of incongruity by investigating the nature of the clutterer's thought process, and then apply the findings to his abnormal utterance.

Thinking Too Quickly

Let us carefully examine the supposition that a clutterer thinks faster than he is able to speak. If we interrupt a clutterer who has reached an articulatory dead end because of what appears to be an attempt to speak as quickly as he is thinking, and ask him to state his thought slowly and clearly, we find that he is still unable to proceed with facility. Either he has no clear thought to express, or he has several indefinite and amorphous ideas.[3] Therefore it is not so much an accumulation of thoughts that speeds him on, but vague and tentative ideas. Froeschels (77:31-33) calls them thoughts that are "unripe for speech." These "germs of thought" occur to the clutterer and he is driven to express them instantaneously. However, coordinated speech requires an intermediate step—a more or less concrete mental formulation of the embryonal thought. Hence the

19   Just how much preparatory thought one needs to be able to speak well is a very difficult point to investigate. In the symposium *Thinking and Speaking*, ed. G. Révész (Amsterdam: North-Holland Publishing Co., 1954), various authors tried unsuccessfully either to delimit the two entities or to prove that both functions are basically the same. In our opinion it is the psychological juncture at which thought becomes speech which is the most important point to consider in this respect. J. Hughlings Jackson (see Search Item No. 2) tried to approach this point in a very suggestive manner, but it does not seem to have been followed up since. Important reference books about thinking, like W. E. Vinackre, *The Psychology of Thinking* (New York: McGraw-Hill Book Company, 1952) and J. S. Bruner, J. J. Goodnow, and G. A. Austin, *A Study of Thinking* (New York: John Wiley & Sons, Inc., 1956), only speak of the one or the other shore of the river, as it were, but do not attempt to build a bridge between thought and speech in action. In the next chapters we shall explore some avenues which might help to clarify this problem in the future.

clutterer does not think faster than he can speak. Rather, he omits a necessary part of the thought process.

Thinking Too Slowly

If thought in preparation for verbal communication is conceived of as an orderly process of clarifying ideas, then clutterers think too slowly for a normal speed of speech. In addition to the pauses in search of a concrete thought for expression, there are gaps while the clutterer searches for a particular (often commonly used) word. His limited knowledge of gram-

3 We use *idea* here to denote a less structured product of mental activity than a *thought*.

mar also slows his thinking. Lack of accentuation leaves long
words without integration, and these words are then misac-
cented, mispronounced, misspelled, and often even misunder-
stood by the clutterer himself. The tachylalia (excessive rapidity
of verbal utterance) manifested by many clutterers worsens the
effect of slow preparatory thought, often rendering speech gro-
tesque. As a result an intelligent clutterer may appear considerably less intelligent than he actually is.

Unorganized Thinking

We can conclude that a poorly integrated and incomplete
thought process, rather than the rate of speed of thought, is a
factor in cluttering. The clutterer's haphazard and tentative
thinking in preparation for speech reflects his general approach
to all undertakings. This is the basic characteristic of cluttering and hence one of the prime targets of therapy.

INNER LANGUAGE

In normal speech, verbalization does not seem to take place
until the speaker has a clear thought to express; he can inhale
the necessary amount of breath to pronounce the length of the
sentence he intends to speak. Thus the normal speaker does
not run out of breath, nor is he left with an excess of breath
(75). In addition, the first notes of his speech melody indicate
the length of the coming sentence or phrase—another sign of
well balanced forethought. Normal speech, then, conveys to
the listener the impression that the speaker knows what it is
that he wants to express and is able to transform his thought
into spoken words with facility. The clutterer's speech lacks this
inner harmony. One of the most basic characteristics of cluttering is a lack of clarity of inner formulation, and as a result,
delivery is hackneyed, haphazard, and studded with moments
when the clutterer seems to lose the thread of thought com-

pletely, or to forget what he has said or the next word to be spoken. We can say, then, that normal speech reflects inner order and cluttering is the mirror of inner disorder.

Many speech pathologists, and most notably Schilling (*184:*-204-46), have studied internal speech—the phase which precedes oral delivery. Most investigators have limited their observations to the motor aspect of internal speech—that is, to the subtle, inaudible speech movements that some people make as an act of preparation for actual speech or when trying to grasp the meaning of a written text, as K. Goldstein (*86*) has described. However, this is part of the preparation for speech only in those individuals who have a motoric disposition.

At this point we have to consider an important but neglected study of the types of imagery. G. Ballet (*12*) enumerates and describes three basic types, discovered by his teacher, Charcot: visual, auditory, and motor-kinesthetic. A normal person employs all three types in varying degrees, but can be classified as a visual, auditory, or motor-kinesthetic type, depending upon which is predominant. Learning and recall can best be achieved when the individual employs his predominant type of imagery in a given task.

We believe that there are three additional types of imagery: smell, taste, and touch. Smell, taste, and touch probably play a larger role in childhood than in adulthood. We can assume, then, that a painter's imagery is predominantly visual, a musician's predominantly auditory, and an athlete's predominantly motor-kinesthetic.

In performing a highly skilled movement the individual generally recalls his previous execution of the same movement, and this is dependent upon kinesthetic sense. However, there is also a purely motor type of functioning in which movements are performed automatically, without recall or imagination of past performance. When imagery (visual, auditory, kinesthetic, smell, taste, or touch) precedes performance, it insures the reliability of the performance. The clutterer's speech process,

however, is a rather automatic performance. Clutterers seem
to need to exert mental effort even to formulate the idea of the
sentence they are about to verbalize, whereas normals apparently perform this inner formulation without conscious effort,
as a function of their predominant type of imagery. Even the
most intelligent clutterers (cluttering is not indicative of lack
of intelligence) are apt to remark spontaneously that they are
often surprised by something they say, being unaware of having
entertained the thought before saying it. Speech (and other
complex acts) performed without the stabilizing effect rendered
by previous imagery of the act can be called *abstract* action, as
opposed to *concrete* action, in which imagery is involved.

Clutterers, then, can be said to be abstract speakers. D. A.
Weiss (*221*:252-62) has shown that they often demonstrate "im-
mediacy of speaking," i.e., their speech is not mediated by imagery and deliberate formulation, but proceeds with a "jump"
from a void in thought to full verbal expression. Some patients
become aware of this void in later years and are frightened by
it. One patient describes abstract speech as follows: "When I
give a speech or participate in a discussion of a complex subject, I feel at first as though my mind is empty. At a certain
moment something seems to tell me 'Go on, it is ready!' Then
I start to speak and sometimes surprise myself with what I say."
Other intelligent patients report similar experiences.

Few speech pathologists have studied the imagery of clutterers. Froeschels and Jellinek (*80*:956-58) and Froeschels and
Kallen (*81*:1162-63) obtained contradictory results. Froeschels,
who did most of the research on the subject, concludes that
clutterers do not have any one predominant type of imagery.
Hence they omit a vital step in the process of speech. They do
not formulate. As a result, their speech delivery (an abstract
action) is uneven or jerky, and often aggravated by tachylalia.

Godfrey Arnold (*7*:82-95) notes the interesting fact that clutterers are often disposed toward abstract sciences. This seems to
be more than the coincidental application of the same word.
One of my patients reported: "I like theoretical mathematics—

just the principles. But I hate 'clerical' mathematics with all the detailed computation and formulas to remember."

It is not possible at this point to prove that clutterers lack a predominant type of imagery. There are tests designed to elicit information about the known types of imagery, but no method has been devised for proving the absence (total or partial) of a type of imagery. Of necessity the material discussed in this chapter is based on clinical observation and patients' reports.

20 For the classical way of testing imagery in general, the book of R. Baerwald, *Psychology of Imagery Types*, 2nd ed. (Leipzig: J. A. Barth, 1928 in German), is unsurpassed. F. Galton, *Inquiries into Human Faculty and Development* (New York: E. P. Dalton, 1908) is an important historical document and M. R. Fernald, "The Diagnosis of Mental Imagery," *Psychological Monographs*, XIV (1912), 1-169 yet a quite useful approach. W. B. Swift in "A Psychological Analysis of Stuttering," *Journal of Abnormal Psychology*, X (1915), 225-35 tried to prove that stammering is due to a lack of visual imagery; this was contradicted by J. M. Fletcher, "The Mental Imagery of Stutterers," *Journal of Abnormal Psychology*, XII (1917), 34-43. The latter also tried to refute C. S. Bluemel's theory (25) that stammering was due to a temporary loss of auditive imagery. C. F. Diehl and N. C. England, "Mental Imagery," *Journal of Speech and Hearing Research*, I (1958), 268-74, tried to re-introduce the approach of mental imagery to the field of speech pathology.

READING DISORDERS

One of the most characteristic symptoms of cluttering is reading disability. Virtually all clutterers manifest a reading problem, and in fact, such difficulties may occur as a pathognomonic indication (decisive diagnostic symptom) when certain other circumstances make the diagnosis uncertain.

The dyslexia of the clutterer may appear at all age levels. In young clutterers we may find that poor reading is a result of having learned to guess at (or having memorized) the text; the root of the problem here is that certain letters of the alphabet have not been learned. Consequently spelling problems in reading and in writing may persist through and beyond the highest grade of school attended. This is closely related to the clutterer's lack of attention and results in his ignorance of many words with high-frequency-usage scores. In addition the clutterer reads longer sentences in the very same manner in which he speaks, i.e., in short phrases. This causes him to lose the trend of thought. Moreover, he is so much accustomed to reading in this superficial manner that he considers it quite natural to be unable to retain the content of what he reads.

The quality of the clutterer's oral reading clearly demonstrates that he does have difficulty in reading, but we must not attribute this difficulty, then, only to poor delivery. His silent reading is just as faulty. In fact, we might infer that his reading aloud is somewhat better because the verbalizing enforces a slower pace and more regularity than silent reading, which imposes no limitations.

The clutterer, as a rule, does not actually read; he skims. When he reads aloud we may observe him trying to glimpse the end of the sentence before he has reached the middle, or looking back at the beginning because he has lost the trend of thought. There is generally not much repetition, even in oral reading; rather there are misreadings in the sense of prolepsis (anticipating a sound before its turn), postposition (pronouncing a sound after its turn), metalepsis (confused sequence), and other seemingly pure articulatory deviations. Even more important are the dyslectic errors based upon inexact reading and fanciful guessing, resulting in the substitution of similar-sounding words, the meaning of which may be completely different from that of the text. An intelligent, seventeen-year-old clutterer produced the following substitutions within five minutes of reading aloud: *these-there, when we see-we have seen, artists-art, bias-basis, works-words;* he also omitted repeatedly short words like *when, we, and.* Often, as a result of the clutterer's attempts to guess what will follow, toward the end of longer sentences he will drop words (elipsis) or add his own words, often entirely unrelated to the meaning of the text. At this point he is not reading, but completing sentences from his phantasy. These fanciful substitutions may be logical, in terms of the sentence, or they may completely distort its sense. As a rule, when a word with which the clutterer is not familiar appears, he will substitute a similar word.

21   Many cases in which dyslexia is the presenting symptom belong properly to the domain of Central Language Imbalance. B. Hallgren's book (96) gives a good general view of the problem. L. Bender (17:155-76) gives deep insight into such cases in which she also finds a maturational lag of language. K. de Hirsch (49:257-61 and 50:235-50) analyzes the dyslectic problems of cluttering children from both theoretical and practical viewpoints.

Analysis of the clutterer's mistakes indicates that the vocabulary of even an intelligent clutterer is markedly restricted. One of my patients, a Ph.D. candidate, was unfamiliar with such words as *impetuous, intrepid, stultified, wily,* and *speculatively.*

It follows logically that the clutterer's silent reading would demonstrate similar gaps if we were able to test it. Many of our patients report that on rereading a book they find that they have completely "forgotten" certain pages, as though they had never read them. In fact, we find that they never did read them! At these points, unknown to them, their attention had lapsed almost to the zero point. One subclinical clutterer (he had corrected himself spontaneously) reported that when reading a particular novel he was surprised to note that he could foresee all the turns of the plot. He read more than half of the book before realizing that he had actually read it before. Correction of this constant wavering of attention is one of the major therapeutic problems in cluttering.

We must not be deceived if the clutterer does not evidence this reading difficulty immediately. Sometimes it will take four to five minutes before his attention starts to waver, and he presents us with an ever-increasing and more colorful bouquet of reading errors. This fact is important in diagnosis. An additional proof of the clutterer's inattention is his unawareness of his mistakes and his denial of even having committed them, in which case he is honest, but twice mistaken.

Specific and isolated dyslexia—in which there is a deep-seated inability to read despite concentrated effort—should not be confused with cluttering. The reading of the typical clutterer is superficial, but his ability to read is not entirely lacking. If we control his wavering attention his reading will improve spontaneously, although generally for a short time only. Painstaking exercise, however, can enable him to manifest his reading potential—a potential which is lacking in the dyslectic.[4] In short, the quality of the usual dyslectic's reading is commensurate with his lack of potential, whereas the clutterer usually does not fulfill his reading potential.

WRITING DISORDERS

The clutterer's handwriting is characteristic of his generally reduced motor skill, his rather formless imagination, and his disregard for the reader. Occasionally we find the repetitions of his speech (full syllables and short words, or simply repeated traces) in his writing as well.

Klara Roman-Goldzieher (*176*:116-39, *177*:28-39, and *178*:-41-58) devoted several articles to this problem. She discusses the general characteristics of the clutterer's handwriting, i.e., smudginess, formlessness, and irregularity, and also the specific characteristics, i.e., repetitiveness, frequent transpositions or omissions of letters, and frequent revisions. She also studied the handwriting of clutterers as opposed to that of stammerers, concluding that the two disabilities are closely related and that cluttering is the more basic of the two. It would be interesting

22   In 1916 J. S. Greene (87) described a case which he called *agitophasia* (agitated speech) *with agitographia*. He cites essentially the same symptoms as Roman-Goldzieher and Schulmann.

to study the development of handwriting during the course of treatment for cluttering. Our hypothesis is that it would improve, but would lag behind the progress in verbal delivery. Based on these considerations, it would seem advisable to cor-

4 This should not sound a pessimistic note for the dyslectic, as he, too, can develop his potential.

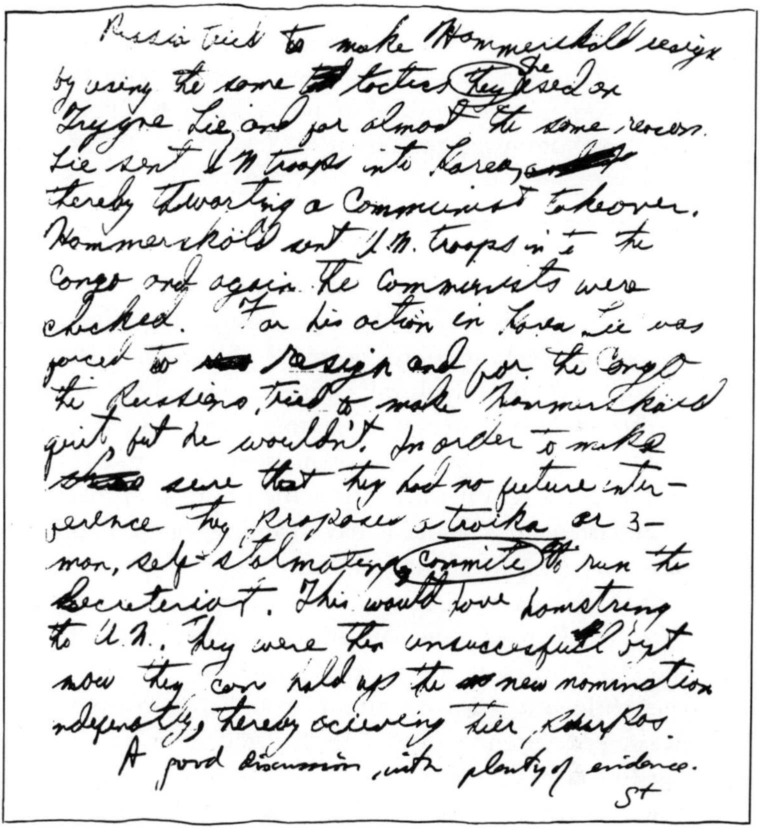
Russia tried to make Hommerskold resign
by using the same tactics they used on
Trygve Lie and for almost the same reasons.
Lie sent U.N. troops into Korea,
thereby thwarting a Communist takeover.
Hommerskold sent U.N. troops into the
Congo and again the Communists were
checked. For his action in Korea Lie was
forced to resign and for the Congo
the Russians tried to make Hommerskold
quit, but he wouldn't. In order to make
sure that they had no future inter-
ference they proposed a troika or 3-
man, self-stalmating commite to run the
Secretariat. This would have hamstrung
the U.N. They were then unsuccessful but
now they can hold up the new nomination
indefinately, thereby acieving their purpos.
A good discussion, with plenty of evidence.
St

Figure 4. Handwriting of a 14.3-year-old clutterer with "very superior intelligence" but rather poor spelling ability. From K. Roman-Goldzieher (*178*).

rect handwriting jointly with the speech in the treatment of cluttering.

In some cases of cluttering errors in handwriting—and even in typewriting (*208:*1-5)—are pervasive enough to suggest that they are symptomatic of dysgraphia. We must consider this question in the light of what has been said about dyslexia. The clutterer is capable of much better performance when he focuses his attention upon the task. It should be noted, too, that the boundary limits between the specific dyslexias, dysgraphias, and cluttering are sometimes fluid. The most complete and lucid discussion of this problem, together with the results of psychological tests, will be found in Klara Roman-Goldzieher's last (posthumous) publication (*178*:41-58).

GRAMMATICAL DIFFICULTIES

The clutterer's spoken grammar is also notoriously poor. Throughout his speech (but not his writing) there are minor deviations, such as confusion of *he* and *she* and the use of the singular when the plural is indicated. There is often total confusion in the structure of long sentences.

The clutterer's attention span is so short and his concentration so weak that he often gives the impression that his hearing is impaired, or that he is daydreaming, or even that he has a basic disorder in perception. Since we remember only that to which we have paid attention, the clutterer's lack of attention to speech (to his own as well as to others') results in a poor memory of correct grammatical usage.

A child learns correct grammar and usage through the recall of correct sentences similar to that which he is about to utter—not by learning and applying the rules of grammar. Therefore applied grammar is basically a function of attention and memory (*74*). In the case of child clutterers it would therefore seem plausible that there would be some grammatical difficulty. Whether an adult can have a specific "grammatical ability," independent of attention and memory, is not known.

Mostly, however, it is not the ignorance of grammar which interferes with the correct sentences of the clutterer. He might notice grammatical errors—possibly the same ones he commits—in the speech of others. Often, too, he writes more grammatically than he speaks because then he has to proceed with more deliberation. But his sentences become overlong by picking his way at random, as it were, adding one short phrase to the other and, at the same time, omitting to finish a sentence before starting another. Toward the end he might forget how he started and so the grammatical structure of his sentences suffers. Clear thinking leads to well structured sentences. The rather fuzzy thinking procedures of the clutterer lead to a less-than-satisfactory structuring of his sentences.

23   E. Froeschels, "Grammar, a Basic Function of Language-Speech," American Journal of Psychotherapy, IX (1955), 45-53 can serve as an interesting introduction to the psychological and clinical approach to lack of thought clarity. M. Solomon and Gertrude Stein in their "Normal Motor Automatism," Psychological Review, III (1898), 492-514 studied automatic writing while the attention was distracted: the grammatical deviations as well as repetitions show an interesting similarity to cluttering and, at the same time, with the idiosyncrasies of Gertrude Stein's personal style. See also B. F. Skinner, "Has Gertrude Stein a Secret?" Atlantic Monthly, CLIII (1934), 50-57.

During therapy it will be seldom necessary to help his apparently poor grammar. When he learns to speak more deliberately, the better integration of his thought processes leads automatically to better structured sentences.

Unawareness of symptoms

The typical clutterer is unaware of his speech disorder and may even react with surprise when his attention is brought to the problem. Stammerers, on the other hand, are keenly aware of their difficulty and constantly struggle with it. The clutterer's unawareness of his speech difficulty is a specific case of his general lack of self-awareness. He is overly spontaneous, compulsive, unorganized, and often unaware of the consequences of a given act. He is a poor follower, and appears to be a bold leader, but in fact, he usually merely acts without premeditation.

Clutterers are poor listeners, impatient to vocalize only their own thoughts. They are not interested in listening in turn to those of others. This is the reflection of a centrifugal (exteriorizing) attitude that is strong enough to submerge the centripetal (interiorizing) functions—perception, awareness, consideration of others, etc. Thus in speech as in action, the clutterer proceeds with sudden impulsive spurts, uncontrolled by the smoothing influence of a modicum of self-awareness or an appreciation of the needs of others.

The characteristic short attention span may also contribute to weakening the clutterer's perception severely. A. Liebmann (119) suggested delimiting a subgroup of clutterers based on perceptual difficulties. E. Froeschels (73) suspected sensory aphasia in some cluttering children. G. Arnold (7:82-95) considers the poor perception a severe, aphasia-like symptom which he calls *perceptual dysgnosia*. Much research is needed in this area.

RESTLESSNESS AND HYPERACTIVITY

The typical clutterer fidgets by day and is restless even while sleeping, according to Seeman (190). He seems to be alert and interested in his surroundings, but for a short time only, since his focus of interest changes continually. During an interview he is apt to squirm in the chair, occasionally assuming odd positions, to play with objects on the desk, and to gesture more expressively than is warranted by the subject matter. This activity appears to be the outcome of a motor drive, which would also account for the clutterer's tachylalia and "compulsive" talkativeness. Therefore some authors conclude that cluttering is the result of a lesion of the striatum pallidum. In fact, there are many cases of proven lesions of the basal ganglia with restlessness of this sort. The Seeman school assumes that submicroscopical lesions in this area are the cause of the clutterer's hyperactivity. However, when a clutterer is given ample opportunity to satisfy his drive fully, he sometimes turns to a quiet occupation or even to daydreaming. Hence it becomes apparent that there is another determinant of his behavior, namely, his short attention span.

Some child psychiatrists assume that this restlessness or hyperactivity reflects emotional etiology and treat it accordingly.

We believe, on the contrary, that it is a basic constitutional characteristic of clutterers. The clutterer is not aware of his restlessness, but if it is brought to his attention, he will exert effort to control it. After a short time, however, he inevitably forgets his intent and returns to hyperactivity. This is behavior suggestive of the young child's lack of controls, and hints at lack of maturation.

DELAYED SPEECH DEVELOPMENT

In the case histories of many clutterers we find indications that the patient, as well as members of his family, began to speak rather late. We must consider the reason for this delay to be the constitutional (inborn) weakness of their speech disposition. On the other hand, a late start in speaking does not necessarily lead to cluttering. There are families in which children generally begin to speak later than the average age of onset, but who manifest no speech disorder.

In our temperate climate the average age at which children begin to speak is about one year. In warm climates where children develop earlier it may be sooner. In Cuba it seems to be about ten months. D. McCarthy (132:476-581) and others have shown that girls start to speak somewhat sooner than boys and maintain their lead for a long time. This might be related to J. M. Tanner's (202) interesting findings that the bone development of newborn girls, based on X-ray studies, is more advanced than that of newborn boys, other factors held constant. This would indicate that girls are more mature at birth than boys, or more pointedly, that boys are born prematurely in comparison to girls. This fact would explain the greater mortality rate, more frequent morbidity, and slower development of speech in infantile males. It might even shed some light on the question of why there are so many more male than female clutterers and stammerers.

24 H. Schuell (186:277-98) has collected valuable literary material on the differences in physical development of boys and girls.

There are, then, factors of maturation involved in the development of cluttering, unlike the simple delay in families where most of the children (especially the boys) start to speak late but ultimately develop satisfactory speech. In the typical clutterer it is not simply a delay of speech or language functions which impresses us, but the *unevenness* of the development of the various functions. That is, there may be no corresponding retarded development of other functions, which may be average or even superior. Thus an intelligent candidate for a Ph.D. degree might have a surprisingly small vocabulary, lacking even commonly used words. A well known scientist who is editor of a medical encyclopedia might demonstrate grave orthographical errors as well as extremely poor public speech, and an accomplished musician might speak in a monotonous and arhythmical clutter. These are actual cases which we have encountered in practice and which could be multiplied ad libitum.

In cases of delayed speech, in general, the following rule of thumb seems practical: if a child does not speak at the age of two, it is possible that he will develop a speech problem; if he does not speak at three, he will probably develop one (exception: familial disposition); if he does not speak at four, we *have* a speech problem.

In general, there are no indications that minimal and discrete lesions are involved in cluttering. We believe that it is principally a matter of hereditary maturational processes.

ELECTROENCEPHALOGRAPHIC FINDINGS

In 1951 Luchsinger and Landolt (*129*:135-49) were the first to attempt determination of the speech pathology of clutterers by electroencephalographic examination, adding clutterer-stammerers and pure stammerers in later investigations. They found abnormalities in almost 100 per cent of their first cluttering sample. EEG examinations of stammerers were actually begun much earlier, but led to no conclusive evidence except for a higher incidence of abnormalities than in the average population.

25 About the electroencephalographic findings in stammerers, see L. E. Travis and W. Malamud (206:929-36) and L. E. Travis and J. R. Knott, "Bilaterally Recorded Brain Potentials from Normal Speakers and Stutterers," Journal of Speech Disorders, II (1937), 239-41.

Luchsinger and Landolt's initial conclusions were later revised, but the evolving literature—Streifler and Gumpertz (200:344-59), Luchsinger and Landolt (130:12-43), Luchsinger (122:7-64 and 123:183-90), and Moravek and Langova (145:-305-16)—did clarify one rule: there are more irregularities in the EEG records of clutterers than in those of stammerers, whose irregularities in turn exceed those of normals. The relatively small number of patients examined by any one investigator explains the large differences in percentages, but the basic relationship remains constant: clutterers > stammerers > normals. Much depended upon the individual researcher's criteria for what he considered irregular or pathological.

The significance of these results is still questionable. On the one hand the activity of the deeper-lying structures, often considered the possible neurological sites of cluttering (190), does not register, as a rule, on EEG recordings. On the other hand, the evaluation of EEG recordings in general today is a very individual matter except in the case of clearly defined disorders, such as epilepsy. Consequently the definitive evaluation of these

26 We hope that future researchers will heed two warnings: Hallowell Davis (47:825-34) remarked that the brain waves that are registered by the EEG procedure are not identical with the nerve impulse, but are "simply a by-product of activity, like the noise of an automobile." Stojanow and Heidrick (199:13-18) demonstrated the dependence of the EEG upon the grade of relaxation of the individual, and Luchsinger and Landolt (130: 12-43) concluded appropriately that the emotional state should be taken into consideration.

results, which suggest, but do not prove, a central neurological disorder, will have to be postponed until the EEG becomes a more meaningful diagnostic tool. This does not imply that EEG examination should be considered futile at this time. These examinations do contribute important raw material to research and may help to delimit subgroups within clutterers in the future.

27   A very practical introduction to the study of EEG can be found in Hughes' *Introduction to Clinical Electroencephalography* (Bristol, Eng.: J. Wright & Sons, 1961).

HEREDITY

We have found that heredity is a basic factor in cluttering. Nonetheless, only a few systematic studies have been made on this influence. The reasons are obvious: first, as we have said before, only a small percentage of clutterers willingly seek treatment, and second, cluttering has not been included in many statistical analyses of speech disorders. R. Milisen's "The Incidence of Speech Disorders" (*141*:246-66) cites innumerable statistical studies, only one of which (*213*:113-21) includes cluttering. A venerable concept in the Old World, cluttering has yet to achieve status in the New.

It is important first to define what we mean by heredity. In view of the close connection between cluttering and stammering that we have postulated, we shall have to seek a common origin of the two disorders with its roots in heredity.

In the families of ninety-five "pure" stammerers Freund (*71:-*146-68) found twenty-nine stammerers with tachylalia, seven stammerers, and twelve tachylalics—a total of 50.5 per cent of such anomalies. In the families of twenty-six stammering clutterers he found two stammerers with tachylalia, twelve stammerers, and ten tachylalics—a total of 92.5 per cent of such disorders. Freund concedes that tachylalia alone might not have

28   The heredity of stammering has a very extended literature. The student of this problem will read with profit J. M. Wepman, "Familial Incidence in Stammering," *Journal of Speech Disorders*, V (1939), pp. 199-204 and O. J. Graf, "Incidence of Stuttering among Twins" in (*105*).

been a sufficient criterion on which to elicit all the data relative to cluttering. Poor word memory and lack of talent for verbal formulation are elements which the family might not notice, but which are important components of the symptomatology of cluttering.

Our clinical findings coincide with Freund's. In virtually every case, by simply questioning the patient's parents we discover that at least one other member of the family has had a speech disorder. Most often it is the father who exhibits cluttering symptoms, and he is generally unaware that the most offensive aspect of the situation is the mirroring of his own disorder in his offspring.

Confirmation of the heredity theory by unprejudiced investigators is noteworthy. Gedda, Bracconi, and Bruno (83:1-20), in a report on speech disorders in twins, cite a family in which there are male twins, one of which previously stammered and the other continues to stammer; a paternal uncle, the maternal grandfather, and his brother are stammerers. The father, his two uncles, two first cousins, and a second cousin have tachylalia (the three generations consist of sixty-four persons). The authors are apparently surprised to conclude that tachylalia and stammering seem to have a common genetic substratum.

Figure 5 shows a family tree reported by the mother of a stammerer. She was a native of a country (Hungary) where the concept of cluttering (hadarás) is well established in the population at large.

Given the fact that professional speech therapists often overlook cluttering, we can deduce how difficult it is to elicit observations of cluttering from the layman. Nonetheless, we believe that eventually the role of heredity in cluttering will be proven conclusively. Only then will we be certain whether we are dealing with real primary cluttering or with the clutter-like symptoms of a more or less discrete organic lesion.

Present indications point to the theory of preferential hereditary transmission from male to male. There remains, then,

29   Only G. Arnold (8:246-54) indicates a higher incidence of cluttering in females. It is interesting that S. T. Orton (153) finds also a prevalence of females affected with strephosymbolia (confusion and disorder of symbols).

this puzzling question: in what form is cluttering inherited? Are there small foci of degeneration? Are there parts of the nervous system which do not mature sufficiently? If it is a personality trait which is inherited, in what cellular or chemical composition can this be transmitted to the new generation? We have found no pathological anatomy in cluttering cases, and we would expect no gross anatomical findings. These are problems to be solved by geneticists.

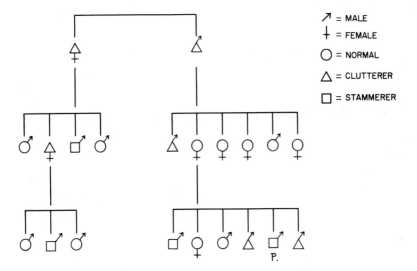

Figure 5. Mixed heredity of cluttering and stammering. Spontaneous report. The grandfather and the great aunt of the proband (P) were clutterers. There were "many other clutterers" in the family. No report beyond the two described branches was available. In this part of the family there were two female clutterers, five male clutterers and four male stammerers. The proband was a clutterer until 13 years of age and then developed stammering.

THE PSYCHOLOGY OF THE CLUTTERER

There is an almost complete dearth of information concerning the systematic psychological examination of clutterers.

Klencke *(114)* characterizes clutterers as carefree, careless, and lacking in persistence and sense of responsibility. The majority, indeed, seem to have some of these characteristics in common. They are generally of pleasant temperament and do not take life's problems very seriously, including, alas, their treatment. They have a short attention span, which precludes their carrying a grudge, persisting in a given task, or keeping a promise for long (although their promises are sincere and their transgressions sincerely regretted). They tend to be overactive, but change pace occasionally and change their mind frequently. For instance, a young clutterer might change toys frequently, or request food urgently but leave it untouched and then wonder because his lack of direction is questioned. In more mature clutterers we are apt to find personal untidiness, disorder of possessions, and lack of punctuality. Clutterers often sit restlessly, squirming or assuming unusual positions—each for a short time. Impatience is their basic characteristic.

In summary, we can say that we may expect to find most or all of these characteristics in the typical clutterer: impatience, superficiality, casual acceptance of life, lack of consideration of the consequences of a given act or for other people, and a short temper which is easily placated. For example, Demosthenes was called *argans* (the violent).

The development of human intelligence and speech, according to Froeschels,[5] proceeds from a wholistic to a progressively more detailed outlook. An individual affected by Central Language Imbalance deviates from this line of development. His attention to detail never develops to the degree shown by his normal contemporaries, and consequently the clutterer exhibits abnormally childlike behavior, reactions, and often even appearance. Rorschach test results in our clinical experience seem to reflect the clutterer's wholistic outlook, including more *W*'s

[5] "Structure of Speech and Stuttering." Lecture in the New York Society for Speech and Voice Therapy, January 9, 1963.

(whole perceptions) and fewer *d*'s (small details) than would be
expected of an individual of the given age. However, to inter-

> 30   The psychological testing of forty stammerers with the Rossolimo and
>   Rorschach tests by E. Ingebregtsen, "Some Experimental Contributions
>   to the Psychology and Psychopathology of Stutterers," *The American
>   Journal of Orthopsychiatry*, VI (1936), 630-50 shows among the ten
>   characteristics at least eight which we associate with cluttering. Attempts
>   at a systematical psychological testing of clutterers will be found in K.
>   de Hirsch (*48:*231-48) and K. Roman-Goldzieher (*178:*41-58). Dumke
>   and associates (*57:*155-69) used for this purpose the rather promising
>   color-pyramid test described by R. Heiss, *The Color-Pyramid Test of Max
>   Pfister* (Bern: Huber, 1951), in German. R. W. Rieber (*170:*87-88) started
>   to explore the dependency-independency problem in clutterers and stam-
>   merers. In our opinion, the perseveration discussed by C. E. Spearman
>   (*195*), J. Eisenson (*59*), J. Eisenson and Pastel (*61:*626-31), P. T. King
>   (*112:*10-12 and *113:*346-57) have much bearing on cluttering. K. de
>   Hirsch, "The Oral Language Performance of Premature Children and
>   Controls," *Journal of Speech and Hearing Disorders* (in print) starts a
>   very promising research which tries to establish the testable criteria of
>   immaturity in speech.

pret these results as stemming from emotional problems alone
is probably incorrect, although it is often done. Rather, it is an
organopsychic situation (Bleuler), recently elaborated upon by
Schick (*181:*235-50). We feel that a basic disposition of hereditary nature lies beneath the symptoms.

Almost without exception clutterers are poor listeners, more
interested in exteriorizing their own viewpoints and feelings
than in hearing those of their interlocutors. In other words, the
clutterer generally takes the lead in a dialogue, disregarding the
other's thoughts and feelings. This behavior is possibly a factor
either of impatience or of weak sensory reception. In conversing
with a clutterer one can expect to be annoyed by his callous-
ness and inconsideration. However, we must keep in mind that
this behavior is not hostile—it is simply childlike egocentricity.

Because the psychological disposition of the clutterer differs
from that of the stammerer, our theory that stammering usually
develops from cluttering might appear contradictory. Van Riper (*211*), however, postulated correctly that stammering itself
changes the individual's character. The psychological character-

istics of the clutterer, then, can be regarded as *primary* (imbedded in the individual's basic disposition), while those of the stammerer are *secondary* and due to the individual's reaction to his constant struggle with speech. Before our theory on the relationship between cluttering and stammering was formulated, we worked with a group that we called *happy stammerers*, none older than fourteen years. Today we would label them *clutterer-stammerers*. They spoke quickly between stammering blocks and were not distressed by their stammering. It follows almost as a rule, then, that the speech symptoms parallel the psychological disposition of the patient. If cluttering symptoms predominate, lightheartedness prevails; if stammering symptoms predominate, brooding prevails. These are merely clinical observations, however, which need systematic psychological research to substantiate them.

The difference in the psychological disposition of the clutterer and the stammerer brings to mind H. Freund's (71:146-68) question of why some clutterers become stammerers while others do not. The key to the answer will perhaps be found in the child's environment. Wendell Johnson's theory that those who are labeled stutterers by their elders may be precipitated into (secondary) stuttering—stammering—appears to be valid.

31   W. Johnson, "A Study of the Onset and Development of Stuttering" in (105) may be reinterpreted in terms of cluttering-stammering.

Some clutterers, particularly adolescents, become angered by their persistent failure to achieve grades commensurate with what they and their teachers believe to be their potential. These children are labeled *underachievers*. The typical clutterer, unaware of his speech problem and generally a poor reader, simply does not know how to overcome his underachievement. He is a diligent student at times, but his performance does not improve accordingly and he becomes worried, frustrated, truant, and unmanageable at home. He may finally be referred to a psychiatrist because of apparent "emotional difficulty." We cannot, of course, always assume that these symptoms are not of a purely emotional nature. We must bear in mind, however, that the basic problem of a large number of these youngsters stems from their Central Language Imbalance. When we see an underachiever, we should look for cluttering.

The erratic behavior and school performance of the typical clutterer often leads to short-tempered and even explosive behavior at home. This is occasionally the presenting symptom in some teenagers whose speech problem does not seem too important. (We saw several such cases who came for a psychiatric consultation because of their domestic difficulties.) If our diagnostic interview elicits symptoms of cluttering, we explain that the patient's irascibility is mainly due to despair about his constant failures both in domestic discipline and academic performance. The real reasons for his failure are his lack of concentration and unawareness of mistakes.

Such an explanation might lead to an almost immediate pacification of the situation at home; the patient starts behaving less desperately, because now he understands his predicament. A similar situation exists among the juveniles in mental hospitals, among which we (224) were able to find the greatest amount of manifest clutterers. Their diagnosis ranged from primary behavior disorder, when under sixteen years of age, to psychopathic personality when beyond this age. They are mostly severely retarded in writing and reading too. The typical restlessness of the individuals affected by Central Language Imbalance and their constant failures in school drive them into truancy and bad company. In such cases we have to consider that their behavior disorder—and later psychopathic behavior —are *secondary* to their Central Language Imbalance. They should not be punished but treated in terms of their basic problem.

Compensation

Another group of clutterers worthy of special mention consists of cases of self-corrected Central Language Imbalance. These clutterers exert great effort to achieve self-correction, but generally continue to manifest a few symptoms. They are likely to become compulsively and rigidly perfectionistic through over-compensation in their speech or in other areas. When excessive rigidity in speech is encountered, one must always investigate the possibility of overcompensation. A well known professor at the University of Vienna can be cited as an example. He was the editor of a highly esteemed scientific journal, and was punctilious in his work. His speech was mournfully slow, his voice monotonous, and he exasperated his listeners with compulsive perfectionism in every detail. I was surprised to find that his office, on the contrary, was in complete disorder. The riddle was solved the very first time that I heard him lecture. He spoke slowly enough, but with constant repetition, interruption, and circumlocution. In fact, I later discovered that he was reputedly one of the worst lecturers at the university. Except for the slow rate of speaking, he manifested all symptoms of cluttering. Although he was unable to control his cluttering when speaking publicly—the most difficult task for clutterers, according to Liebmann (*119*) and Freund (*71*:146-68)—he could control it when simply conversing. Furthermore, he was able to compensate in matters relating to his journal. The total disorder of his office, in our opinion, indicated his cluttering tendencies, in more than one sense.

This example will serve to illlustrate another point. Contrary to the impression of superficiality given by their speech and behavior, the few existing psychological studies of clutterers reveal them to have at least average intelligence. Central Language Imbalance belongs to the basic matrix of the individual, predating his dialogue with the world and influencing both his emotional and intellectual development. Although this definition might seem to indicate a flaw in the individual's basic makeup, it should not lead to the erroneous conclusion that the clutterer is thus necessarily inferior in general. He has some specific weaknesses, especially in his processes of communication, but nonetheless he may be capable of unlimited intellectual achievement.

Numerous examples can be cited of great personalities in world history who were clutterers. We may point to Demosthenes, to whom an aged admirer said: "You speak just as Pericles did." Luchsinger (*126*) quotes Gregorius von Nazizanz as witness that Justinian, the great lawgiver of the Middle Ages, was a clutterer. There also was Bismarck, one of the most important statesmen of nineteenth-century Europe, and in our own time, Winston Churchill. Although it may be premature to cite specific traits associated with cluttering in Churchill's personality, his listeners will have noticed his "light stutter." Each of these contributors to world history viewed his world wholistically, and was not deflected by exaggerated attention to small details. Perhaps, then, they excelled because of, rather than in spite of, their Central Language Imbalance.

Clinical observation indicates that most cases of self-corrected Central Language Imbalance are women. Often they demonstrate compulsive perfection in their personal grooming, but divulge their actual disposition by one or two flaws, such as dirty gloves or shoes in need of repair, in an otherwise impeccable appearance. They are tense, driving, restless, and constantly harassed by the fear that they have forgotten something. Their speech is quick and staccato. These characteristics are indicative of their effort to compensate for a low level of organization.

One might question, then, whether or not these compensation characteristics might result from the therapy for cluttering. The answer is—emphatically—that they would not. Self-corrected clutterers achieve partial and sometimes appreciable success, but it is their disproportionate effort which yields these characteristics. The therapist's primary goal, in contrast, is to increase the patient's power of concentration and to lengthen his attention span. When these measures are successful, less effort and rigidity occur in day-to-day activity, communication, and social relations.

These observations permit us to deduce the importance of

recognition of the primary component of a genetic disposition in the psychological makeup of the clutterer. This disposition affects his perception, retention, and reproduction. In view of the far-reaching effects of Central Language Imbalance upon an individual's general performance and of the much greater incidence of Central Language Imbalance that we have heretofore suspected, the need for psychological testing and examination of clutterers is apparent. Testing would probably result in the delimitation of subgroups.

Subgroups

Liebmann (*119*) divided clutterers into two subgroups: the motor group, in which accelerated speech and articulatory deviation are the predominant symptoms, and the sensory group, in which difficulty in finding necessary and appropriate words is the predominant symptom. (This breakdown corresponds roughly to the usual subdivisions of aphasia.) D. A. Weiss (*216:*-1-19) has added a third subgroup, in which general difficulty in formulation is the predominant symptom (corresponding to transcortical aphasia). A fourth subgroup is occasionally included, consisting of clutterers whose speech is exaggeratedly slow and interspersed with drawn out *ah-ah-ah*'s or *a-a-a-*'s, especially in public speaking. This group is a logical inclusion in a breakdown of cluttering because the interjections are a result of chronic difficulty in word selection and/or formulation.

The four subgroups may appear to be distinct on first clinical observation. On close inspection, however, it is generally found that each case of cluttering that we see possesses certain symptoms associated with each of the four subgroups. Therefore, it is preferable instead to view the criteria for differentiating subgroups within cluttering as facultative symptoms of cluttering. In this way the significance of the interrelationship of all the symptoms and the basic factors underlying them is not concealed by the process of subgrouping according to predominant symptoms.

The only valid reason for ascertaining which of the many symptoms is predominant in a given case of cluttering is for the purpose of directing therapy to relieve the most obvious symptoms first. Carrying therapy to its logical extreme would involve work on every channel of communication—obviously an impractical measure in a typical case of cluttering. Various authors (20, 42, and 44) suggested learning foreign languages, because the clutterer speaks better in them than in his native tongue; dancing which educates the rhythmical sense; acquiring social graces which lead to a more controlled and balanced performance, and the like. This calls to mind the practice of ancient Greeks and Romans who raised their noble sons with the sole purpose of excelling at public speech. We must be content to eliminate the most obvious symptoms and thus improve the clutterer's processes of communication to the point of acceptability.

The influence of environment, of course, cannot be discounted. Observation in foreign countries reveals that in warm southern countries (socially outgoing) there is evidence (42) that more cluttering than stammering exists, while in the cold north we find more stammering than cluttering. Negroes and the temperamental Latins of Europe, as well as South Americans, also seem to show relatively more cluttering. The incidence of stammering and cluttering in the northern as opposed to the southern United States would make an interesting and enlightening study.

Organic cases, including those whose lesions are congenital, must be considered as a separate entity, despite the similarity of their speech symptoms to those of the clutterer. In addition to proof of organicity there is another differentiating criterion: organic cases are generally shy, withdrawn, quick to take umbrage, resentful of criticism, and generally unsure of themselves—as opposed to the devil-may-care attitude of the typical clutterer. Systematic investigation will eventually determine the reason for diametrically opposed psychological characteristics in these two groups, both of which manifest similar symptoms as far as their verbal delivery is concerned.

SUMMARY OF SYMPTOMS

The manifold symptoms of cluttering can be arranged in the same way as the classical scheme of the various kinds of aphasia. This should not mean that we necessarily equate these two disturbances. We only consider it as a useful manner of systematizing the possible disorders of language.

The excessive speed and the articulatory deviations, as well as the restlessness, in general, can be considered as motoric (expressive) failings. The repetitions, drawling, and interjections are the manifestations of difficulty in word finding. The weakness of perception and unawareness of disturbance, along with the reading and writing difficulties, belong to the sensory (receptive) side of the ledger. The grammatical difficulties seem to stand astride the line which separates (or unites) the expressive and receptive realms of speech. The poorly integrated thought processes and the gaps of inner language can be paralleled with transcortical aphasia. Lack of rhythm and of musicality bear resemblance to amusia.

The frequently delayed speech development, the strict heredity, and the electroencephalographic findings seem to situate cluttering among the organic disturbance. On the other hand, we can observe an immediate—although short-lived—improvement and even disappearance of all symptoms when the clutterer concentrates his attention upon the task at hand. This circumstance places the weakness of attention into a central position so far as the problem of cluttering is concerned.

The majority of symptoms of cluttering are *facultative,* i.e., often present but not necessarily so. Only a few are *obligatory,* i.e., symptoms which are *always* manifested and which clinch the diagnosis. The obligatory (pathognomonic) symptoms are: (*a*) short attention span and its corollary, poor concentration, (*b*) lack of (complete) awareness of the disorder, and (*c*) an excessive number of repetitions in speech. We expect that future research might reveal a reduced capacity of perception as an obligatory symptom. The most common facultative symptom is reading disorder, especially in reading aloud. Overhurried speaking, although quite frequent and most impressive to the listener, is only one of the facultative symptoms.   ~~~

CLUTTERERS GENERALLY REVEAL SOME UNIQUE PECULIARITIES DUR-
ing the first interview. Most young clutterers are unaware of
their difficulty, often state that they do not understand the reason for the examination, and even consider the interview an
inconvenience imposed upon them by their parents. Adult clutterers often cite as their only complaints the difficulty in public
speaking or their irritation at being asked frequently to repeat
because they cannot be understood. They are unaware of further difficulty.

The most conspicuous elements of cluttering, such as excessive speed, repetition of syllables, and the difficulty patients
often label *getting stuck,* can often be elicited in the taking of

3 *diagnosis*

a careful case history. The therapist should immediately clarify
what the client means by his "getting stuck": does it refer to
a blocking with muscular effort (stammering component) or to
inability in finding the necessary word in time (the cluttering
component)?

One of the most definitive indications of cluttering is that
the clutterer's speech is poorest when he is in relaxed situations,
with his family or friends, and that it improves under tension,
as in the initial interview. When he is under pressure the clutterer tries to control his speech and may even succeed in con-
trolling his symptoms completely for a time. Therefore, the
clinical examination will require an amount of time sufficient
to enable the patient to relax and, as a result, to begin to speak
in his usual manner. This rule of thumb is applicable: if the
parents' complaint is "stuttering" and the patient manifests no   *63*

signs of a speech disorder at first, cluttering is indicated. In an occasional case the general picture will not be unfolded until subsequent visits, but cluttering can usually be diagnosed during the initial interview, with additional symptomatic details uncovered as therapy progresses.

The therapist begins a typical first interview with short questions requiring short answers, in order to allow a tentatively diagnosed clutterer to retain control of his speech. Next the therapist introduces a topic of particular interest to the patient. The subject matter should be such that the patient can discuss it with a minimum of interruption or questions. Hobbies, aspirations, television programs, and books are but a few suitable topics. As the discussion becomes more relaxed the patient lessens his control and, if he is a clutterer, reveals more and more symptoms, whereas the stammerer might improve through adaptation.

The second phase of the first interview is reading aloud, one of the most effective diagnostic techniques, since clutterers find great difficulty in exerting even a minimum of control over their symptoms when involved in the process. A simple text is most efficacious because the goal is to achieve relaxation and hence this minimal control. Difficult texts require increased concentration which results in greater control, and our task is to evoke the symptoms. Material written by the patient, a letter for example, which is familiar and therefore unchallenging to him, is often most revealing. A clutterer will first misread the minor elements of the text, such as word endings, prepositions, and short words. As he continues there is hesitation, repetition, and even changes of the entire end phrases of sentences. Instead of reading the text, the clutterer substitutes sentence endings out of his imagination. He guesses as he reads.

In most cases at this point in the interview the diagnosis will be fairly conclusive, and to support it the therapist can question the patient or his parents about areas other than communication in which clutterers typically perform poorly. Is he careless? forgetful? unaware of the consequences of his actions?

The final phase of the interview (s) is the discussion of treatment. Since the typical clutterer is unaware of his difficulty, a problem is likely to arise in convincing him of the necessity for therapy. When logic is of no avail—and it rarely, if ever, suffices —the therapist must try to determine whether the patient is satisfied with his speaking and reading ability. The clutterer will often acknowledge that he has some doubt about these abilities, but that they hardly seem to warrant the effort required for therapy. Although the amount of effort and attention required for the successful treatment of cluttering is greater than for that of other speech problems, and the clutterer is not highly motivated, therapy should not be begun unless the therapist is certain of the patient's cooperation. Thus, demonstration of the disability and its effects on general performance is an important function of the first interview.

Given the failure of logic and the unwillingness of the patient to expend the effort demanded by therapy, as a last resort the therapist can play a tape recording of the patient's speech. This will often supply convincing proof of the disability. The examiner's speech should also be recorded to prevent suspicion of a faulty tape or machine. Listening to himself can be a traumatic experience for the clutterer because he suddenly becomes aware of the extent of his disability and hence can no longer remain unconcerned. He must be assured that his full cooperation and a sufficient amount of therapy will lead to success.

DIFFERENTIAL DIAGNOSIS

In true cluttering there is practically always the presence of a hereditary factor and the absence of neurological symptoms. The first step in differential diagnosis, therefore, is exclusion of cases of symptomatic cluttering, i.e., the cluttering-like symptoms that result from neurological disease. Any kind of brain lesion—traumatic, infectious, tumoral, etc.—can upset language function and produce cluttering-like symptoms. In most cases of adult aphasia the disorder called *stuttering*, in our opinion, is actually symptomatic cluttering. We rarely encounter real stammering in adult aphasia, although it is occasionally seen in children who become aphasic at a very young age. It should be interesting to determine whether there is a definite age beyond which no real stammering develops in aphasics. In our experience we have not known stammering to develop in childhood aphasics after the age of nine or ten. We have carefully scrutinized all reports of later onset and find that they are actually the aggravation of a latent stammering which had existed previously.

Epidemic encephalitis produces the syndrome most similar to fully developed cluttering. The hurry and precipitation ("drivenness") which characterizes the movements of these people is particularly noticeable in their speech. In addition to overacceleration there are articulatory mishaps, such as anticipation, postpositioning, irregular jumbling of the sounds of a word, telescoping, and often paretic hoarseness. The difficulty seems to be primarily motoric involvement, but no systematic testing of sensory perception in epidemic encephalitis has yet been undertaken. The pathological substrate consists of lesions in the basal ganglia (the clusters of gray matter at the base of the brain), which participate in the articulatory process. Foremost among the ganglia are the globus pallidus, the putamen, and the nucleus striatus; the entire system is called the *striatum pallidum*. Lesions of the striatum pallidum are considered to be the cause of disturbances of articulation in epidemic encephalitis. Some authors, like P. Schilder (*183*:668-70) and M. Seeman (*190*), even consider stammering to be a neurosis of the striatum.

The striatum pallidum seems also to be the principal organ involved in bulbar (more appropriately *suprabulbar*) disorders. The exact role of the various formations in this region is not known. Pathologic anatomical findings are scarce and not unequivocal, and the personal conviction of a neurologist determines the nucleus he considers affected in a given case. The paucity of pathologic anatomical information, however, does not adversely affect therapeutic intervention. The striatum pallidum may also be affected by all kinds of meningitic, encephalitic, and traumatic lesions, such as in punch-drunk boxers (*157*:82-83). In these cases there is no precipitation, but on the contrary, there is diminished speed, with articulatory deviations resembling those of cluttering. Dysarthria may also evolve.

Symptomatic cluttering is frequently found in the mentally retarded. The hurried, repetitious speech and occasional vowel stops of the mongoloid are characteristic (*36*:34-37). Most of the mentally retarded do not develop true stammering. Development of true stammering seems to come as the result of concentrated effort to improve the fluency of speech, and this requires a keen memory of past failure. This is beyond the capability of the severely mentally retarded. Thus the "stuttering" mental defective is generally a symptomatic clutterer.

Symptoms resembling those of cluttering may gradually appear in people who have become totally or partially deaf after the development of speech. The voice becomes higher pitched and often soft. Articulation is indistinct and sometimes slightly slurred. As opposed to clutterers, who have never developed adequate speech, the deafened have lost auditory control of their speech.

The main differential diagnostic task consists in delimiting cluttering from stammering. This will be treated in the next chapter.

THE RELATIONSHIP BETWEEN CLUTTERING AND STAMMERING CAN be considered the most important single relationship in the field of speech pathology. The occasional appearance of the two disorders together was noted in the early literature by Hunt (*103*), Gutzmann (*91*), Treitel (*207*:578-664), Scripture (*187*), and others, but no systematic relationship was hypothesized. On the contrary, the two disorders were thought to be totally independent of one another. In some texts they were cited together as *disturbances of the rhythm of speech,* but nevertheless they were discussed as unrelated phenomena. In all of the literature

4 *cluttering and other disorders*

major importance was accorded stammering (stuttering), and, if anything, only token mention was given to cluttering.

Freund and Weiss discovered a meaningful relationship between cluttering and stammering. Freund (*70*:1446-57) noted that both speech impairments often appeared simultaneously in family groups and hypothesized that a hereditary element was involved. Weiss (*215*:1-4) noted that after the strong tonic symptoms of stammering were cured, symptoms of cluttering appeared.[1] He concluded that since stammering generally started with cluttering-like symptoms and left a cluttering-like residue when cured, it was probably an outgrowth of cluttering. Investigators in many countries later corroborated Freund and

[1] H. Gutzmann (*91*) noted this fact in 1893, but drew no conclusions from it.

Weiss' theories; this possibility, therefore, can be considered a consensus of the investigators of cluttering.

Since cluttering and stammering are associated with opposite psychological characteristics, the theory that at least the majority of stammering cases are based on pre-existing cluttering may appear to be implausible at first. Colombat *(44)* and Kussmaul *(116:*581-893) wrote in the early literature that stammering is aggravated by tense situations or close attention to the speech process and that cluttering, on the other hand, is aggravated by relaxation and improved, at least temporarily, by increased attention to the speech process. The list of opposite psychological and situational characteristics of clutterers and stammerers was augmented by Freund *(70:*1446-57), Weiss *(216:*1-19), and most recently by Arnold *(7:*82-95). We shall consider the most important typical differences:

	Cluttering	*Stammering*
Awareness of disorder	Absent	Present
Speaking under stress	Better	Worse
Speaking in relaxed situation	Worse	Better
Calling attention to speech	Better	Worse
Speaking after interruption	Better	Worse
Short answers	Better	Worse
Foreign language	Better	Worse
Reading a well known text	Worse	Better
Reading an unknown text	Better	Worse
Handwriting	Hasty, repetitious, uninhibited	Contracted, forced, inhibited
Attitude toward own speech	Careless	Fearful
Psychological attitude	Outgoing	Rather withdrawn
Aptitude (academic)	Underachiever	Good to superior
EEG	Often diffuse dysrhythmia	Usually normal
Goal of therapy	Directing attention to speech details	Diverting attention from speech details

On the whole, the effort to control the speech process is beneficial to the clutterer and detrimental to the stammerer. This contradiction was at the root of the initial resistance of numerous investigators to the theory that cluttering and stammering are interrelated.

At the turn of the century Gutzmann (92), Hoepfner (100:-16-57), and Froeschels (75) noted that the majority of instances of stammering are preceded by a phase of effortless repetition, prolongation, hesitation, and self-correction, which they called *physiological stuttering*. Freund (70:1446-57) appropriately changed this term to *physiological cluttering*. Almost all children between the ages of two and five manifest this nonfluency, which is considered a normal phase of development during which expressive capacities (vocabulary, grammar, formulation) lag behind the desire to communicate. As his ability to express himself increases (apparently in conjunction with increasing familiarity with words and partly due to the maturation of the nervous system), the normal child's nonfluency disappears. The minority of children, however, continue to manifest symptoms of nonfluency regularly and beyond the normal ages for physiological cluttering. Some children manifest these symptoms markedly from the very beginning of verbalization. It is not unusual to hear it said that these children think faster than they can speak. In fact, as we have mentioned earlier, this was Hippocrates's theory of the basic cause of stammering. As we have seen, it is not the speed of thought, but the desire to speak which outdistances their capacity for expression. The mother of one of these children might define the situation by saying, "Johnny stutters a little." Typically this group is livelier, more restless, less considerate of others, less orderly, and more quick-tempered than their contemporaries. They seem to be at odds with their utterance, but completely undisturbed by this fact.

Bluemel (27:187-200) endeavored to establish a distinction between the physiological stumbling of the developing child (nonpathological) and the somewhat pathological unevenness of speech delivery which could lead to serious complications. He called the latter condition *primary stuttering*. The child, he emphasized, is unaware of his deviation and should not be scolded or punished for it. Many theorists objected to the concept of primary stuttering because it cannot be defined precisely. In addition, we object on the ground that since primary

32   The arguments against the concept of primary stuttering can be found in P. J. Glasner and F. D. Vermilyea, "An Investigation of the Definite and Use of the Diagnosis, 'Primary Stuttering,'" *Journal of Speech and Hearing Disorders*, XVIII (1953), 161-67.

stuttering indicates merely the possibility that stuttering (stammering) will develop—although many of these children never develop secondary (real) stammering—the use of the term *stuttering* would appear to be undesirable before the fact.

Regardless of the effects of nomenclature, however, the clinical fact is that at the inception of the vast majority of cases of "developmental stammering" (73), i.e., stuttering which develops in early childhood, there is a special phase which bears the characteristics of cluttering. This is evidenced by the child's *lack of awareness* of his repetitions, hesitations, and prolongations. He does not recognize that he shows a faster tempo of speech than that commensurate with his capacity for expression. These cluttering symptoms are still manifested when the stammer has developed completely (at least in the initial phase of development). In addition, in stammering as opposed to cluttering, there are the misdirected efforts of the patient to suppress his symptoms. Even in adult stammerers bold and careless spurts of speech often alternate with self-conscious and fear-ridden blocks. In recent literature these patients are referred to as *clutterer-stutterers*. We prefer to call them *clutterer-stammerers*.

Henry Freund (71:146-68) emphasized that stammerers might accelerate their speech in order to finish quicker because they were afraid of running into trouble. He called it *secondary tachylalia*. Several early authors voiced the same opinion, and also some of the stammerers we have treated confessed to the same feelings. On closer observation, however—which is possible only during systematic therapy—we could note that it was, in fact, the same primary tachylalia which characterizes many clutterers. On the one hand, the stammerers (we saw) were disposed to speak the quicker the less they were afraid of running into blocks (relaxed situation), especially after being relieved through therapy from the major part of their impediment. On the other hand, when we tried to call their attention to the hurried character of their speech, they appeared to be quite surprised and said that they always felt that this rate of speaking was natural and appropriate. When we had occasion to point this out to a stammerer, who told us in the beginning of therapy that he was hurrying out of fear of blocking, he ruefully admitted: "I really had that impression at the time; now I know that it was only an excuse."

In the adult stammerer his extreme self-consciousness and his morbid attention to the articulatory details often lead to disappearance of the vestiges of cluttering. When treatment is effective, the lessening of apprehension in turn lessens blocking, and cluttering symptoms reappear, according to Gutzmann (*91*) and Weiss (*215*:1-4 and *216*:1-19).

In summary, cluttering is usually observed before the stammering develops; it persists in the early stages of stammering until suppressed by the patient's efforts; and it reappears when stammering lessens. These facts led to our conclusions on the basic relationship between cluttering and stammering diagrammed in Fig. 6.

Speech disorders which the general public categorize as "stuttering" actually might belong to any one of three categories: (*a*) pure cluttering (Fig. 6, left), (*b*) pure stammering (Fig. 6, right), (*c*) cluttering-stammering (Fig. 6, center). Cluttering-stammering is the most frequent phenomenon, at least among individuals who seek professional help.

Based on our therapeutic experience (no observation can be considered conclusive without ample therapeutic experience), we have become doubtful of the existence of pure stammering, i.e., stammering not based on cluttering. The patient may con-

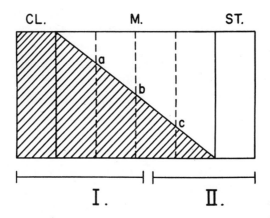

Figure 6. Schema of the relationship between cluttering and stammering. Cl = cluttering; M = mixed (cluttering-stammering); St = stammering. I. Therapy should start with the treatment of cluttering. II. Therapy should start with the treatment of stammering. From Weiss (221).

sult us during the phase when cluttering is suppressed and deny that his stammer was preceded by lack of speech coordination. But we have never observed a case in which cluttering symptoms did not emerge after the stammering symptoms had lessened. One patient noted ruefully at this stage of treatment: "Before therapy I was so busy overcoming difficulties with one or another word that I never noticed that my thoughts were not ready in the first place."

Esti Freud [2] reported that of a patient group consisting of veterans who started to stammer suddenly after war traumas (shell shock, etc.), each individual admitted that he had had some degree of speech disorder before his accident. (The veterans were assured that this information would be held confidential so that it would not affect their compensation claims.) It is more difficult to determine the quality of the premorbid speech of children whose stammering is reported to have de-

[2] Personal communication and remark in the discussion at the XIth Congress of the International Association of Logopedics and Phoniatrics, London 1959.

veloped suddenly after fright. For this reason we cannot conclusively disprove the existence of "pure" stammering.

It has been said jokingly that our procedure converts stammerers into clutterers. There may be a kernel of truth in the accusation. Since we consider cluttering to be the basic disorder, it is essential that treatment of stammering should consist, in part, in the treatment of the cluttering component if therapy is to be permanently successful.

With regard to the general plan for therapy, pure clutterers and pure stammerers should be treated according to the demands of their basic difficulty. Clutterer-stammerers, the majority of those who seek treatment, require more specific and careful planning. When the cluttering component predominates (Fig. 6, a), therapy should begin with treatment of cluttering, since the possibility exists that this procedure may eliminate all symptoms. Specific treatment of the stammering component should be begun only when it becomes apparent that it is necessary. When the stammering component predominates (Fig. 6, c), therapy should begin with treatment of stammering, but it will always be necessary to treat the cluttering component when the stammering blocks have lessened. When cluttering predominates, if treatment for the stammering component is applied prematurely, the effect will not be detrimental. When stammering predominates, and treatment for cluttering (increasing attention to articulatory details) is applied prematurely, however, stammering can be aggravated.

A novel approach is likely to be mistrusted, especially when there have been no foreshadowings of it in the literature. As long ago as 1870 James Hunt (103) wrote: "Although cluttering and stammering are essentially different, they are frequently combined in the same individual. . . . My experience leads me to believe that cluttering, more or less pronounced, generally precedes stammering in children." [3] Treitel (207:578-664) wrote

_____

[3] J. Hunt used different expressions; we substituted our own nomenclature.

in 1892 that "a clutterer whose speech is so hurried that he gets stuck, becomes a stammerer only when he gets afraid of speech. ... It is often difficult to distinguish whether a patient is a clutterer or already a stammerer." The leading scientific schools in Europe during the first decades of the century described stammering as developing from a state of imbalance of speech in the young child. This imbalance was renamed by H. Freund (71:-146-68) as *physiological cluttering*. Bluemel's conception of *primary stuttering* is consistent with this point of view. Scripture in 1912 (187) is more specific, noting that "cluttering is usually combined with stuttering" and "sometimes produces it." In our view, all these authors can be considered as precursors of the idea which we are proposing in this chapter.

Our own point of view is that cluttering is the principal if not the only basis of developmental stammering. Occasional concurrence with this idea, which is considered extreme by many authors, has appeared in the literature (108, 109, and 169:109-13). Other researchers in this field, among them Liebmann (119), Hudson-Makuen (102:1070-73), Nadoleczny (149:-1076-1183), Froeschels (79), Freund (71:146-68), Pichon and Borel-Maisonny (159), Boome (30:126-30), Arnold (6:25-45), de Hirsch (51:3-9), Bloodstein (23:3-69), and Van Riper (211), go so far as to admit that a certain percentage of incidences of stammering may develop from cluttering, but these authors also include other precipitants, such as fright, psychic trauma, and environmental influences.

Nevertheless, we have been forced by our long and intensive study of these disorders to conclude that the great majority of stammerers, if not all of them, show a developmental sequence. They begin as clutterers and become stammerers or both.

In this respect it might be interesting to mention some remarks which seemed to be rather cryptic at their time, but might be judged as prophetic as far as our views of the relationship between cluttering and stammering are concerned.

L. E. Travis (205:95) wrote in 1931: "The stutterer, like most

other types of speech defectives, reflects a certain lack of maturation of the central nervous system which either does not afford
integration of the highest neurophysiological levels involved in
speech or predisposes these levels to disintegration by various
types of exogenous and endogenous stimuli."

M. D. Steer (198:13) in 1937: "In other words, stuttering
might be defined as a function of maturation involved in speaking. And therefore adults who stutter, do so because of a condition of arrested development in the speech mechanism."

C. Van Riper (210:185) in 1937: "It is interesting that the
symptoms he (Bluemel) termed primary are precisely those
which we found to be common to all adult stutterers."

In this context we also cite the often expressed views by
Nadoleczny (149:1076-1183) to the effect that stammering is frequently based on a hereditary weakness of the disposition to
speech.

This series could be prolonged indefinitely, and it would be
interesting to know how these authors would relate their earlier
pronouncements to the latest developments.

Our theory that at least the majority of stammering cases
are the result of the patient's misdirected attempt to overcome
the basic cluttering component integrates numerous independent theories and therapeutic procedures, some of which seemed
to be contradictory heretofore. Instead of a cross-sectional view
of cluttering and stammering, this approach affords a longitudinal view of both the development and reduction of pathology.
As a result, our theoretical evaluation and therapeutic intervention can correspond to the appropriate phase of the disorder.
We can cite as an example of seemingly contradictory theories
of the Viennese school of Froeschels, which advocated diverting
attention from the articulatory details in stammering, as opposed to the Berlin school of Gutzmann which advocated more
attention to articulatory details. Both schools found that their
theories were corroborated by practical experience. In the light
of the newer longitudinal view there is no contradiction; both
measures are applicable, but each to a different phase of pro-

gression or regression (cf. Fig. 6). In our opinion the results of therapy based on the theory of the interrelationship of cluttering and stammering give clinical support to the validity of the theory.

CLUTTERING AND DYSLALIA

Cluttering is often complicated by dyslalia, the misarticulation of certain consonants.[4] The most affected consonants in cluttering are the same as those of the other dyslalics, i.e., the sibilant sounds and the [r] sound (rhotacism), this latter being often confused with [l], or changed to [w] or [j].

Demosthenes also showed, besides his impetuous speech which made him appear to have been a clutterer rather than a stammerer, this same kind of [r]-[l] confusion according to Plutarch (162). Aetius (1), a sixth-century physician, noted the combination of delayed speech, hasty delivery, and the [r]-[l] confusion as a characteristic combination. After describing this observation, which is quite remarkable for his time, he recommends the panacea of his epoch: cutting the frenulum of the tongue.

As we have seen, the clutterer is more unaware of his own articulation than is the average person. He is also less painstaking with his delivery and often motorically underendowed. Many clutterers do not show any dyslalia when speaking slowly

33   Seeman and Novak (191:170-76) tried to prove by having their subjects repeat simple syllables that the clutterers are not inferior in their ability of articulation.

and deliberately, but appear to be dyslalic when speaking in their usual hasty and careless way.

Some clutterers, who are completely unable to articulate certain consonants correctly, appear able to imitate immediately or to learn quickly the correct articulation of a missing con-

4 The inability to articulate any vowel of one's mother tongue seems to be generally indicative of a dysarthria due to brain lesion.

sonant, yet be unable to use it in free-flowing speech. The carry-over from exercises to everyday speech is notoriously poor in the clutterer and this constitutes their main therapeutic difficulty in general.

The dyslalias and their therapy will be treated in this series by J. A. Carrell. Here we want to add only that, in our experience, it seems usually to be advantageous to start out with the treatment of dyslalia if dyslalic behavior is present in the clutterer. Such treatment forces the clutterer to pay attention to the details of his speech and therefore slows down the rate of his delivery. We would, therefore, treat the misarticulation first.

CLUTTERING AND VOICE DISORDERS

The clutterer's voice is usually a bit louder than normal and only in a minority of cases is it lower, sometimes approaching the level of a murmur, especially at the end of the sentence. This is a result of his unawareness of the acceptable vocal intensity needed in conversation. Consequently, we often find the signs of overstrain of the voice, a hoarseness of various degrees. This can happen even when the usual volume of the voice is below the normal level, because the voice is then not relaxed, but rather "suppressed." In our experience the voice of the typical clutterer lacks the clear ring of the normally relaxed voice. The particularly strong drive and impatience of the clutterer might be considered as the main source of this deviation.

The rather ruthless manner in which the clutterer treats his voice might appear in children as wild noisiness. They are often quicker and louder than their contemporaries. The same attitude might exert a particularly negative influence at the time when a certain carefulness is necessary, such as the period of pubertal change of the voice. Some of our most resistant voice cases are those of the mutational falsetto—when the mutational disorder appears concomitantly with cluttering.

34   For the occurrence of disorders of the pubertal voice in cluttering, see
      D. A. Weiss (220:126-59).

The clutterers also often show a certain nasality of the kind which is best described as the nasal twang. It resembles open nasality (hyperrhinolalia), but is associated with the constriction of the upper pharynx. Depending upon one's point of view, this can be considered as either an articulatory or voice deviation. S. Blanton (22:156-72) mentioned it in a case which showed the typical symptoms of cluttering and also other therapists [5] noticed it quite frequently. Here we have also the signs of the hyperfunction which is due to the great drive of the clutterer, along with his unawareness of mishandling his own voice.

Voice disorders and their treatment will be considered in another volume of this series (A. Murphy, *Functional Voice Disorders*). It is pertinent to point out here our experience in cases where a serious voice disturbance was connected with marked cluttering. As the voice exercises and their carry-over into everyday speech require more persistence and concentration than the untreated clutterer is able to muster, it is preferable first to treat his cluttering.

[5] C. Van Riper, Personal Communication.

CLUTTERERS ARE INATTENTIVE TO THE DETAILS OF THE SPEECH process and heedless of their speech in general. Any therapeutic approach to cluttering, then, must be based on calling attention to one or more sharply defined details of the speech delivery. The carelessness that clutterers manifest in spontaneous speech, and often even during therapy may well be exasperating to the therapist. Klencke *(114)* characterized clutterers as "sanguinic"—choleric of temperament, flighty, careless, and without persistence.[1] Stulli *(201:367-72)* concluded that "there is no way other than to beat them with a stick." Today's approach is quite different; the results are different too.

The therapist should keep in mind that the clutterer is often

5 *therapy*

unable to evaluate his own speech and therefore does not understand what it is that the therapist is demanding of him. Only careful and patient explanation, as well as occasional imitation of the patient's delivery and the use of tape recordings or transcription, can indicate to him what is wrong. This must be done with patience and firmness. The therapist should ask himself constantly what element in the clinical picture seems most disturbing or in most urgent need of correction. This element will change constantly as therapy progresses. However, the therapist must be conservative in considering previous or seemingly successfully treated problems, such as excessive speed or monotony of voice, as having definitively been mastered. These symptoms pertain to a basic disposition, and hence tend

[1] Klencke labeled them "thought stutterers" and "temperament stutterers."

to recur if neglected, or when the patient is particularly care-less. Therapy for cluttering, therefore, requires a complex bat-tery of exercises and activities, the application of which must be adjusted constantly to the needs prevalent in the individual case. The therapist must be just as alert and attentive as he hopes the patient will eventually become as the result of the therapy.

The therapeutic approach, which is directed àt any given time to one or two (never more) elements of the total picture, should remain fairly constant. Frequent change of approach in an attempt at immediate improvement results only in frantic experimentation. No single element holds the key to the solu-tion of the entire problem of cluttering. Frequent changing of the therapeutic approach in an attempt to isolate a single causal element will confuse the patient and might indicate to him that the therapist lacks confidence in his own procedure. The treat-ment of each element can be likened to the slow driving of a long nail into hard wood. If the nail sits fairly well, another should be begun, but the first nail must not be forgotten. Treat-ment of cluttering is a long and tedious process for the patient as well as for the therapist, and it should not be begun before it is ascertained that the patient will cooperate fully and as-siduously. The stammerer suffers enough to ensure a degree of cooperation, but since the clutterer is largely unaware of his dis-order, only painful failure as well as serious confrontation and consideration can induce him to undergo protracted treatment.

An additional incentive may be that as a corollary of this treatment a rewarding increased attention and concentration span develops. Younger patients report consistently that their academic performance improves. In general we prefer not to note this fact until the patient reports it spontaneously, but sometimes it is beneficial to point out this fringe benefit in an attempt to increase cooperation. The patient's cooperation and the therapist's ability to maintain unflagging interest in the therapy are decisive factors in a favorable result.

It will be noted, on the other hand, that many therapeutic

considerations and procedures, which were applied in the past in the treatment of "stuttering," will find their place in the treatment of cluttering. Although the differential diagnosis and the close relationship of cluttering and stammering were not consciously known, the therapeutic empathy (understanding) of the older experts in speech pathology preceded their theoretical insight. They felt instinctively what the patient needed. Their practical procedures show that they frequently recognized the necessity for reorganizing the thinking and speaking habits of their patients in a manner which corresponds to our own view concerning cluttering. However, if this procedure was successful with some patients, all the other patients were treated in a similar manner, notwithstanding their belonging to another phase of pathological development of the disorder. Hence the occasional successes and paradoxical failures of any one-sided therapeutic procedure. In our experience, this longitudinal view of therapeutic considerations gives us a better and surer grip on the treatment of the overwhelming majority of patients.

Before describing the various therapeutic procedures, we must consider an additional factor. In cases of pure cluttering, as in cases where cluttering appears with other disorders, constant attention to articulatory details can do no harm, *except when cluttering is co-existent with severe stammering*. As long as the spasmodic blocks of stammering predominate, strict attention to the details of speech will do more harm than good. How far the therapist can proceed with the treatment of a cluttering component in stammering cases, therefore, must be determined only after careful evaluation.

The reader might properly conclude that when we attack any one of the elements of the cluttering disposition, others may improve simultaneously. Similarly, in the following exercises it will be seen that when any one element of cluttering (excessive speed, lack of attention or concentration, neglect of details, etc.) is brought under control, some of the others will improve. It should be noted, therefore, that most exercises will also serve purposes other than the specific one mentioned in the subtitle under which they appear. This illustrates that it is not any one of these symptoms which lies at the root of cluttering, but rather a faulty attitude toward communication in general.

There are many exercises which improve cluttering immediately, but which are effective only in the presence of the therapist. That is, their effect is not carried over into spontaneous speech. Included here are the exercises which we have found to have the most transfer effect. D. Bradford (*33*:59-65) notes that many patients reach a plateau of improvement after some therapy. This phase should not be mistaken for ineffectual therapy, but calls for further systematic treatment.

SPEED

The oldest form of therapy in our field is probably the simple advice to speak more slowly. Excessive speed not only worsens delivery, but also prevents the correction of mistakes. In the long-range treatment of clutterers, however, the advice to speak slower is insufficient. It might improve immediate performance temporarily, but establishment of the new habit of speaking in a tempo commensurate with the all-around verbal capacities requires more pervasive measures. It is very difficult to get these patients to slow down their rate by exhortation alone.

Syllabization

Syllabization consists of requiring the patient to speak in slowly pronounced syllables, giving each syllable an equal time allotment. This method has been used from the inception of speech therapy. Its many advocates note that it is a boring and tedious procedure, although efficacious to a degree. Its principal limitation is the resulting lifeless manner of speech, which becomes unbearable not only to the patient, but also to the therapist after a short time. However, syllabization is a useful demonstration to the patient (who is always impatient) of the degree to which he deviates from the normal speed of speaking. Therefore it is a practical way of beginning treatment when excessive speed of delivery is the prime difficulty.

Rhythmical Tapping

In fact, rhythmical tapping should be termed *tapping in measure,* since the tapping on the desk with every slowly pronounced syllable does not allow for any variation in time. It is a reinforcement of the syllabization exercise, allowing the patient greater control of his speed of delivery. There may be difficulty at first in coordinating the spoken syllable with the tapping—exemplifying the typical clutterer's difficulty in integrating various simultaneous activities. He might speak in syllables and tap haphazardly, or tap regularly and speak irregularly. (The normal speaker would have to make a strenuous effort to simulate the lack of coordination shown so clearly by the clutterer.)

When coordination of syllabized speaking and simultaneous tapping has been achieved, reading aloud may be attempted. Following this we proceed to spontaneous speaking, first in short sentences in answer to simple questions, and then in longer conversational sequences. The therapist must empathize with his patient in order to know how long he can proceed with this exercise before it becomes too boring for the patient. (The therapist's own boredom should not be a consideration.)

M. Colombat (de l'Isère) (*44*) used the metronome to regulate syllabization and to improve the clutterer's poor rhythmical sense. Other therapists too report that they utilize this method.[2] We have found tapping on the desk more satisfactory because it allows for small variations which make the patient's delivery more lifelike.

2 Robbins (*173*:331-43) mentions that the procedure was used as early as 1750.

Simultaneous Reading Aloud

This procedure, originated by A. Liebmann (*119*), was designed to help the stammerer. However, as we have seen, there
is no sharp line between the treatment of cluttering and that of
stammering. In this procedure the therapist and the patient
read a simple text simultaneously. The therapist imposes a
slow speed, permitting variation and rhythmical accentuation
of syllables. In order to ascertain whether the patient begins
spontaneously to follow the therapist's lead, the latter should
lower his voice slowly and imperceptibly until he is no longer
leading the patient. The accomplishment of spontaneous reading in an acceptably slow manner is an important step forward.
These exercises, which Marland (*136*:242-45) and Bradford (*33:*
59-65) referred to as *shadowing* exercises, do not overtax either
patient or therapist, and are useful in the early stages of therapy.
However, in our own experience, they do not decisively influence the quality of the clutterer's spontaneous speech.

READING

Most clutterers are poor readers. In some cases speech therapy
should be preceded by specific reading therapy. Most often,
however, poor speech habits seem to be the primary cause of
poor reading, and the following exercises might serve to alleviate both problems simultaneously.

Reading, especially reading aloud is, according to Pick (*161:*
136-52, 216-29), the "function nearest to speech." There are
strong cross-connections between reading and speech, and in
cases of cluttering much help can be derived from well conceived reading exercises.

Letter Reading

The clutterer tends to scan a text superficially—taking quick
glimpses at the words to come and occasionally looking backward to recheck. Froeschels (*75*) proposed letting him read

through a paper shield in which there is a hole the size of a single letter. As the patient moves the paper slowly across the line he sees one letter at a time and is forced to concentrate his full attention on it. His delivery is thus decisively slowed. In this activity the patient's initial tendency to slide the paper over the lines quickly should be discouraged. Bradford (33:59-65) suggests underlining the final consonants of words, since they are most apt to be slurred, and Serre recommends covering the following lines of text to preclude advance scanning. The length to which the therapist can proceed with this efficacious procedure will depend upon the nature of his authority over the patient.

Letter reading often results in reading without understanding, but this too may be beneficial in that it can correct another problem of the clutterer, namely, changing the written text to correspond to what he imagines it to be, before having read it completely.

A problem arises with predominantly syllabic languages, such as English, where the phonetic worth of a letter can often be determined only after the whole syllable is known (hat-hate, bit-bite, ranger-wrangling, etc.). Therefore, when necessary, an appropriately larger hole can be made for this exercise.

Phonetic Writing

Froeschels (77:31-33) reports encouraging results by using a simple and ingenious form of phonetic writing. It can be learned speedily but cannot be read quickly. The alphabet is based on the terse indications of the anatomical positions of the articulatory organs during the pronunciation of the various sounds. Because of its naturalness and simplicity, patients consider it a game and recite it with corresponding enthusiasm. Any phonetic writing would suffice for this purpose, but rare is the clutterer who knows the International Phonetic Alphabet! The Froeschels system is clear, simple, and calls the patient's attention to many details of articulation. It does not contain all the refinements required by a linguist, but it is sufficiently expressive to serve our purpose.

The clutterer's attention and concentration upon a single letter are generally defective. The following reading exercises prove especially helpful in this respect.

Reading Backward

The patient reads a text backward, not omitting any letter or word. Depending upon the particular language, he may read literally or syllabically, but in any case, he must omit nothing. For example, *He went to town yesterday* might be read *Yad-retseyn-wot ot t-new eh.* The therapist follows attentively. This technique has the flavor of a game which patients often play enthusiastically. It may also be given as homework under the control of an instructed adult.

If the therapist wants to utilize a less taxing exercise or to have the reading proceed in the normal forward direction, he may have the patient read a text in a language with which the therapist is facile, but which is unknown to the patient. The effect will be similar, with but one exception: it is more a chore than a game for the patient, and motivation flags.

It would be relevant at this point to relate an experience which demonstrates the close relationship of the manifold symptoms of cluttering. During a visit to a grade school in Havana a teacher presented to the author an eight-year-old girl who knew the letters of the alphabet but was unable to read correctly or to speak grammatically. Although the teacher considered this to be the result of an impoverished neighborhood, she nevertheless became exasperated when a good deal of effort affected neither the reading nor the speech problems of this otherwise pleasant, cooperative, and slow-speaking girl. We prescribed exercises in reading backward and repetition of meaningless syllables, promising to look into the matter of her poor grammar somewhat later. Both teacher and pupil accepted the proposal enthusiastically, especially since Spanish lends itself easily to literal reading. When after six weeks we wanted to proceed to the second stage of treatment, the teacher reported that both the reading problem and the ungrammatical speech had disappeared.

Copying and Reading Aloud

The patient is required to copy a text and to pronounce each syllable simultaneously while writing it. This procedure may appear to be clumsy, but it has several advantages. First, the patient must read attentively or he will not be able to copy the text. Second, the process of writing makes him more aware of correct spelling, in which he is often deficient. Third, speech is considerably slowed.

We find this procedure particularly advantageous when the patient is unable to attend therapeutic sessions frequently enough. The exercise may be done as homework and the patient asked to present the written result of his effort at the following session.

35   Simultaneous talking and writing in the therapy of stammerers is best explained in J. Eisenson, ed., *Stuttering: A Symposium* (New York: Harper & Row, Publishers, Inc., 1958), pp. 279-80. It was originally designed by Travis and Bryngelson.

Rhythm

Many investigators have stressed the clutterer's lack of rhythmical sense. Arnold (*6:25-45* and *7:82-95*) most notably has advocated systematic rhythmical exercises which consist of recognizing and repeating simple and then progressively more complicated rhythmical structures. Heretofore syllabization exer-

36   A good description of rhythmical exercises can be found in L. Pearson (*156:51-59*).

cises, in a strict metronomical sense, have resulted in a better balance in timing. We personally have not employed such rhythm exercises independent of speech, but believe that they could be beneficial.

Some clutterers in the beginning are quite surprised when asked to accentuate sharply. They have to learn by practical examples what is meant by accentuating and emphasizing. It is as though they had overlooked this point altogether in their speech development. Often even intelligent and well educated patients show a surprising ignorance of where to put the accent even in rather common words. This parallels certain gaps in vocabulary. We insist, therefore, that every time they are unsure about the meaning of a word or about its correct accentuation, they should look it up in the dictionary. No systematic studying of such words is necessary. If a word is looked up four to five times, it becomes rooted in the patient's vocabulary.

Accentuation

Exaggerated accentuation is one of the most incisive approaches we have found (*223*:216-23) in the treatment of cluttering. It consists of placing an exaggerated stress on every accentuated syllable, e.g., YESterday I MET a VERy GOOD FRIEND in TOWN and we HAD a GOOD TIme toGETHer. Bradford (*33*:59-65) uses simple verses as the material for this exercise and recites in unison with the patient. She has the patient tap on the accented syllables. Originally we intended to use this approach as a means of slowing the patient's delivery in a manner more natural than that of pure syllabization, and we have found that it does contribute to this goal. In the performance of these exercises, however, we discovered that often even the most intelligent clutterer is uncertain of correct accentuation and stress. He is forced, thus, to learn correct timing, which in turn improves his delivery. Another fringe benefit is the counteraction to the extreme monotony or stereotypy of the clutterer's speech.

Patients consistently report the efficacy of these procedures in formulating sentences. An intelligent, fifteen-year-old boy said: "When I hit the accents hard, the whole sentence clears up in my mind." This would indicate that timing is important not only for actual delivery, but for the inner formulation of the sentence as well. The sharply emphasized accents seem to form a mold which gives the sentence about to be pronounced a clear outer contour. This mold seems to create an "active void" which wants to be filled and seems to draw in the words necessary to fill the form. Many patients report that if they "hit the accents hard" the necessary words occur to them more easily.

This exercise has the advantage that it is less artificial and more natural. Indeed, it approaches normal utterance. It does not produce lifeless sounds, as syllabization does. On the contrary, the sounds produced are livelier than normal, and the exercise requires a constant and rather exhilarating effort on the patient's part. In general it is our experience in speech and voice therapy that patients tire quickly if they are requested simply to control, to inhibit, and to hold back. They are more likely to cooperate if they believe that they are actively pushing forward. This exercise seems to provide momentum and to reduce ambivalence.

A question might arise as to whether this energetic method of pronunciation would tend to aggravate a co-existing stammering or cause stammering symptoms to reappear in cases where they had been controlled. Our experience has been reassuring. The sudden and sharp release of syllables effected by the exaggeration has nothing in common with the slowly increasing pressure of the spasmodic contractions in the blocks of the stammerer. These exercises do not aggravate such blocks, even when begun before stammering symptoms have disappeared.

Once the patient has mastered the exercises for speech, they should be employed in oral reading. And when they have been mastered therein, the therapist should encourage the use of this manner of speaking for conversation. At this point the resistance against speaking in an "artificial manner" will have to be overcome. Even more important, however, is the problem of overcoming the clutterer's chronic oversight of the concepts and skills he has mastered thus far. As a suggestion we often use such slogans as "hit the accents hard," "hammer away at them," or "speak like an old doctor who wants to explain something very emphatically to his small patient."

We suggest that accentuation consist only of an increase

in the volume of the voice (loudness) and its pitch, but not in the prolongation of the syllable. The first two factors involve boldness and driving activity, whereas prolonging a syllable involves restraint. This differentiation becomes especially important when we treat cases of cluttering and co-existing stammering.

VOCABULARY AND FORMULATION

Reading

The clutterer's inattentiveness to his own speech as well as to that of others leads to surprisingly large gaps in his vocabulary. All reading exercises probably contribute to increasing that vocabulary. Attentive reading tends to correct the spoken sentence. The attempt to recognize the correct spelling and accentuation of lesser known words in the dictionary is helpful and should become common practice. Only in time will the patient become aware of how often he finds errors on even very common words which he had previously overlooked. This reading should be done aloud, slowly and well accentuated, thus contributing also to the regulation of verbal delivery in general.

Poems

Recitation of poems *learned by rote* has many advantages. It increases vocabulary, teaches more refined formulation of sentences, and, if well accentuated, helps to give speech a rhythmical flow. For the latter purpose, poems with strong rhythm should be selected. At first the learning of poetry by rote may appear to be a most difficult task for the clutterer. With practice, however, many become capable of memorizing poetry with even more facility than normals (*221*:252-62).

Repetition of Stories

The clutterer's inability to recount a given even coherently can be combatted effectively by slowly developing his ability to repeat stories, anecdotes, jokes, etc. Even the most intelligent patients are surprisingly deficient in these skills at first. Froeschels (75), who has emphasized this weakness, describes how clutterers overlook not only significant details, but even the main point of the narration. The insignificant details may be mentioned in a "helter-skelter" fashion. Sometimes a phrase is repeated with exactness, only to be followed by a complete blank so far as the progress of the story is concerned. This clearly demonstrates the clutterer's chronic fluctuation of attention.

It will be necessary at first for the therapist to demonstrate how to organize the main ideas of the story, how to ascertain the main point, and how to relate the regular progression of events. During these exercises the patient should be permitted and encouraged to use his own expressions. There will be no transfer effect when the patient merely repeats the therapist's words. Often several weeks elapse before the patient is able to relate a somewhat complicated story in an acceptable manner. However, the achievement of this goal is a rewarding experience for both patient and therapist.

It might be useful here to analyze the progression of two short stories which we often use at this point in treatment.

There once was a tame elephant who lived in India. Every day he went to a nearby river to drink and to bathe. On the way to the river he had to pass through a small village, where he always stopped at a tailor shop and put his trunk through the window to receive an apple or some bread to eat. One day, however, when he stopped at the tailor shop, he was given nothing to eat. Instead, a boy pricked his trunk with a needle. The elephant continued on his way to the river as though nothing had happened. After drinking and bathing he filled his trunk with water. On his way back he stopped at the tailor shop, put his trunk through the window and squirted the boy who had pricked him. The moral of this story is that an elephant never forgets.

A simple enough story, one would think. But ask your cluttering patient to repeat it! He might have the elephant douse the boy without having gone to the river. Or, he might have the elephant go to the river, but neglect to have him fill his trunk with water. Perhaps he would forget the pinprick, or have the elephant retaliate immediately with the squirt of water—all of which may be said at least to demonstrate that the clutterer does not have the memory of an elephant.

For homework we ask the patient to repeat this story (or similar ones) several times mentally and then to relate it again at the next session. Usually he will render a confused version again. We then call his attention to the main point of our elephant anecdote: crime and punishment. It is important first to stress the habitual aspect of the elephant's walk, without which the story is meaningless. When these basic elements have been made clear, the patient may be able to relate the story correctly. It should be noted that the errors enumerated above are by no means characteristic of the least intelligent or severest clutterers. They are simply characteristic of clutterers in general.

When a simple story, such as the elephant fable, can be repeated accurately, we might choose a more complicated one with a strictly progressive sequence:

A peasant and his son walked down the road, leading a donkey, on their way to the market. Presently they met some other peasants, one of whom said: "Look! What stupid people! They are walking when they have a donkey to ride on." So the father got onto the donkey and the son walked along beside them. As they continued down the road they met some other people. One of them said: "What a heartless father! He rides the donkey and lets his son walk in the dust." The father dismounted and the son got on. They continued in this manner until they met some other people, one of whom said: "What a disrespectful son! He rides the donkey and let his father walk on the hot road." Hearing this, the father climbed onto the donkey and both rode. Very soon they met another group of people, and one of them said: "What cruel people! Two men riding on a small donkey!" The father and son did not know what to do. Finally both dismounted, tied the donkey's forelegs and hindlegs together and carried him on their backs. The moral of this story is: this is what happens to people who listen to everyone's advice.

This story requires a rigorous developmental sequence, and virtually no clutterer is capable of telling it at first. The difficulty generally begins with comprehending the moral, i.e., the basic idea of the story. Then, one or another of the various stages of mounting or dismounting the donkey will be repeatedly omitted or confused. The therapist will find it necessary to reduce the story to its basic structure: first, both walk; then the father rides; next the boy rides; they both ride; finally father and son carry the donkey.

The therapist should not attempt to accomplish successful recitation of such a story in one or two sessions. Each story should be the basic theme of several sessions—until the patient learns not only to recite it satisfactorily, but also how to organize the material so that he is able to apply the method to the recounting of a new story.

Innumerable stories in addition to the two analyzed here may be used, and some may be developed to fit the particular need for increasing levels of complication. The therapist should have several stories at each degree of complexity in readiness. If he uses them repeatedly he will know where to expect difficulty and how best to make the solution of the problem understandable and workable for the patient.

This brings us to movies, television programs, books, and articles—on all of which the patient should be asked to report. Generally these reports will contain few and rather disconnected elements of information at first. Gradually the patient will find that he is able to pay closer attention and to remember more of what he has heard, seen, or read. It is not only the recall which is improved, therefore, but also the initial attention and perception. In his narration it is important that the patient *try to formulate the sentence before verbalizing it.* This will be difficult at first. Some patients simply state that they are completely incapable of planning a whole sentence beforehand. They should be encouraged to try, however, using any method which is least difficult for them. The choice of method will depend upon the patient's predominant type of imagery.

Some will move their lips silently (motor type), others will "hear" the words (auditory type), and still others will "see" what they are about to describe or even "see" the sentence in writing (visual type).

37   C. S. Bluemel (25) considered the stammerer as an auditory-motor type who in his moments of troubled speech showed a "transient sensory aphasia." W. B. Swift (see Search Item No. 19) advocated visual exercises for all stammerers.

The interruption between verbalized sentences will be unnaturally long at first, but will become shorter as treatment progresses. When the therapist has evidence that the patient is well enough organized, these exercises may be discontinued. In fact, no one thinks a complete sentence through when speaking normally and fluently. The clutterer, however, must learn to sense when he is not ready to speak and must develop the discipline necessary to stop at such times and organize mentally what he is about to say.

Rehearsal

As we have seen, the clutterer's repetitions, monotony, frequent grammatical confusions, etc. are caused simply because he wants to talk before he knows what to say well enough. He might have a vague and general idea of the content, but this is far from the concrete verbal formulation he needs. Silent rehearsal of the initial verbal formulation in this exaggerated manner will teach him to sense the point at which he can start to speak, knowing that the necessary words will be at his disposal.

Of all the types of imagery the visual one seems to be the most advantageous for the clutterer. Seeing the words and phrases written before his mind's eye before pronouncing them is very useful, but we have no systematic way to educate a specific type of imagery. Occasionally a patient might arrive at the solution which best suits him—depending upon his prevalent disposition to some type of imagery—just by trying "to think before he speaks." An intelligent clutterer-stammerer, after being given this time-honored advice and having passed through some exercises of attention and concentration, surprised us with the following statement: "Now before I speak, I see the words like written on a screen before my eyes. This happened to me sometimes before, sometimes afterwards." He must have been a predominantly visual type to begin with and found this optimal solution spontaneously. (The cluttering component of the patient seemed to be fully controlled at this time, but the stammering component still required much attention.)

The pinnacle of success in story telling—as far as the clutterer is concerned—is the successful telling of jokes. Clutterers are notoriously poor joke tellers. Toward the end of treatment we can lighten the therapeutic sessions by using jokes as material for speaking exercises. A bonus is thus provided for therapist and patient alike. The purpose, however, is a serious one. A well-told joke requires strongly disciplined inner formulation. The degree to which the patient succeeds will indicate how far we have been able to develop one of the clutterer's weakest points—his mental formulation.

ATTENTION SPAN AND CONCENTRATION

Each of the previous exercises used coherent verbal performance or written text as its basis. Number exercises are also useful in the development of a longer attention span and correction of faulty concentration.

Counting Backward

Counting forward is an almost completely automatic procedure. We have verified that it does not affect the electroencephalogram at all. Counting backward, on the other hand, requires a certain amount of concentration. Inability to count backward is sometimes taken as a sign that the patient's attention is reduced, as for example in the beginning of general anesthesia. Somewhat more concentration is required in regressive counting when diminishing by 2's, or by 3's or 4's.

It is surprising to hear a well educated clutterer begin rapidly to diminish by 3's from 100, and inevitably make mistakes toward the end of the series. The errors are unrelated to mathematical education. It does not take much mathematics to enable a person to deduct three from any number. These errors are due to fluctuation of attention, and hence are characteristically found in clutterers. The subtraction exercise, first from 100, later from 200, etc., is most useful for the development of the attention span and of concentration.

We generally begin by subtracting 3 (2 is too simple). As we proceed with higher numbers we notice that deducting 4 is hardly more difficult, since the resulting numbers repeat themselves in a short and regular sequence (6, 2, 8, 4, 0). Deducting 5 is too simple; 6 is also quite simple. The real difficulty begins with 7.[3] Most clutterers fail on the first attempt with 7's and need much practice and homework before they are able to produce a complete sequence correctly. To prevent memorization of the answers (93, 86, 79, etc.) give the patient any number at random in the vicinity of 100, and later 200, as a starting point. The next step will be subtraction of 13 (the numbers between 7 and 13 are not of sufficient difficulty), and then 17, etc. When we wish to make the exercise even more difficult, we can combine two numbers, for instance, deducting 17 and 14 alternately. This exercise is very demanding both of concentration and of attention span. It is interesting to observe that at first a patient may proceed correctly for a time, make a mistake which he fails to notice, and then continue correctly until the next error. Lapses of attention can be mapped out almost exactly in this manner. If the exercise is performed by a child as homework, an adult with a sufficient attention span should supervise. The child himself would not notice his mistakes.

If a patient is intelligent enough, the following aid can be offered for better control when practicing alone: before begin-

[3] In the classical examination of psychiatric patients, failure in the deduction of sevens is considered a sign of depression. There is some logical reason for this. A depressed person is unable to pay continued attention to any task. The clutterer, although far from being depressed, will manifest the same symptom.

ning the exercise he should determine the points where a number ending with zero is arrived at. For example, starting with 200 and deducting 7's, the next number ending in zero (10 × 7) to which he will come is 130, and then 60.

Description of these exercises may make them appear mathematically complex. Actually, however, they can be understood by any normally intelligent person, and an attempt to master them will provide a challenge. Accomplishment of a given series is in itself a source of satisfaction and at the same time proof of improved concentration.

Patients of grade-school and high-school age report consistently and spontaneously that their learning capacity and their marks improve in conjunction with the performance of these exercises. Even a candidate for a Ph.D. in economics and finance reported that as a result of the number exercise his study habits improved. He had begun with a few mistakes when deducting 3's, and many with 7's, but progressed until he was able to master the alternate subtraction of 17 and 14. Subsequently this patient reported that he passed his doctoral examinations in public financing "with flying colors." (He was actually a clutterer-stammerer, with a stammering component strong enough to obscure the cluttering component until the stammering symptoms were somewhat relieved. However, the cluttering component was always evident in his reading.)

It should be understood that these exercises in counting backward are only a sample of what can be done to improve the inconsistent performance of the clutterer. Bradford (*33*:59-65) draws up lists of one-syllable words in several columns and has the patient learn one, then two and three words of each column and repeat them from memory. Beebe (*15*:273-76) uses the material of the syllabic memory test. Meaningless sounds in increasing number of syllables (*po-te, na-le-co, sa-le-po-te-noo*) can be memorized and repeated. This is a slow but rewarding procedure with the advantage of seeming like a game. A wide field is open for the inventive therapist, provided he understands

what he is trying to accomplish. However, he should limit himself to a number of exercises in which he becomes well versed,
in the way that a musician knows his own instrument best.

TREATMENT OF CONCURRENT PROBLEMS

Treatment of Dyslalias

Clutterers often have some dyslalic disorder. Although this
is certainly an additional difficulty for the patient, a dyslalia
can be used in the treatment of cluttering itself. As we have
seen, any procedure that forces the clutterer to concentrate
more intensely on the details of his speech delivery is beneficial.
The treatment of specific dyslalias is a case in point. For
instance, in order to treat a common lisp, or any other misarticulation error, the patient must pay close attention to his articulation, and hence his delivery is slowed. Without going into
the details of such therapeutic procedures, we would advocate
having the treatment of any dyslalia *precede* that for cluttering.
Our experience has been that this sequence constitutes an excellent introduction to treatment. Since many difficulties may
be corrected by the treatment of a dyslalia, fewer and more
specific problems remain to be treated once the dyslalia has
been corrected.

Chewing Method

Although this method cannot be used for the treatment of
cluttering *per se,* we mention it here for two reasons. First, it
is possibly the most useful approach in the treatment of the
principal complication of cluttering, namely stammering, and
also for treating speech and voice difficulties due to pathological
concentration on certain details of phonation. Second, when
efforts to concentrate on the details of speech have overshot
their mark, the chewing method constitutes a strong corrective
in "relaxing" the patient's speech.

Froeschels's chewing approach is based on his conviction that

38   D. A. Weiss and H. H. Beebe, eds., *The Chewing Approach in Speech and Voice Therapy* (Basel-New York: S. Karger, 1950) describes the procedure and its various applications.

the origin of speech was a vocalized chewing, as found today among the aborigines. Hence he considers vocalized chewing movements as being basically identical with speech movements. Consequently, to make the patient "chew" when he speaks or sings might be termed a return to nature—to that kind of phonation which preserves its pristine purity and relaxation, unhampered by cultural pressure. It is said to be the strongest "normalizer" of spastic or otherwise exaggerated speech and voice delivery.

The patient is best introduced to the chewing method in the following manner: after explaining to him that we can exhale soundlessly (as we normally do) and also with vocalization (sonorously), we ask him to exhale both ways in a relaxed and natural manner. The sonorous exhalation should sound as though the patient were breathing (exhaling) normally, but producing a sound as in sighing. Any deliberate change in pitch or volume should be avoided. Next we ask the patient to imagine he has something, such as an apple, in his mouth and to chew it, not politely with closed mouth, but primitively and carelessly, as though munching it vigorously. He is then asked again to exhale sonorously and to chew "like a tired farmer munching an apple before falling asleep." The patient should be able to perform each step automatically before he is introduced to the next.

Next we explain that this procedure is the natural basis of speaking (and singing), and then we begin with simple material, such as counting (chewing the numbers) or a scale (munching the sounds). We have the patient speak, read, or sing progressively complicated material, always keeping "chewing" in mind. We must carefully keep him from imitating chewing by artificial movements and see that he performs an uninhibited, automatic chewing movement. He should chew psychologically as

well as with his mouth, and at least at first discard any inten-
tionality from his speech. Speech requires so little intention-
ality that it is virtually unnoticed by the speaker if performed
in a relaxed manner.

To derive the maximum benefit from the chewing approach
it is essential that the therapist know the method thoroughly.
It is a simple procedure, but one that must be followed exactly. Unskilled "chewers" were the basis for some scurrilous
reports about the method, which we, on the other hand, consider to be the most important single therapeutic procedure in
logopedics and phoniatrics.

As mentioned above, because it is completely opposite to
the therapeutic approach to cluttering (concentration on detail
and strict control of delivery), "chewing" can be used only in
some specific complications of cluttering.

Voice Problems

Clutterers often have voice problems that are generally overlooked in the mutational deviations of the male voice (*220:*126-
59). The treatment of voice disorders is considered in another
volume of this series, but an important warning should be mentioned here about the timing of the treatment in cases of cluttering and coexisting voice problems. Contrary to what we have
said above about the treatment of dyslalia, in cases of cluttering
and coexisting voice disorder the cluttering should be treated
first. If the voice problem were to be considered first, the
patient would not have enough discipline and self-control to
follow the instructions and perform the exercises necessary to
improve his voice. Many failures in the treatment of voice
disorders occur because the underlying cluttering is overlooked.

Summary of the Speech Therapy

We have described the therapeutic approaches and provided
some specific exercises which may be applied to alleviate cluttering. It should be understood that many of these exercises

have proved useful in the treatment of speech disorders which fall into other categories, especially aphasia and similar organic disorders. This does not necessarily mean that all of these disorders belong to the same order. Rather, it calls attention to speech itself as a particular function with its own laws, rules, and necessities. If the function is disturbed in any particular manner, restoration of full harmony and integration must be achieved according to the basic rules of speech in general.

PSYCHOTHERAPY

Occasionally the speech therapist—or any other therapist—feels helpless when his utmost efforts to aid his patient have failed, and it is then that the question of the necessity for psychotherapy arises. Until the end of the 1930's cluttering was considered a rather hopeless therapeutic task. Current methods are more successful, but the question of psychotherapy, nonetheless, should be considered here.

Essentially, any therapeutic procedure has a psychotherapeutic element as a component. The injection which would seem to indicate that the physician knows precisely how to treat a given illness, the bitter medicine which might indicate to the patient that he has endured the suffering necesssary for recovery, and foremost of all, the personality of the therapist who, in the eyes of the patient, assumes the role of a benign father figure or wears the witch doctor's cloak of awesome superiority—all of these elements are psychotherapeutically important. Similarly, the technical advice given in correcting a person with a specific speech disorder, especially when the advice proves helpful, may be considered symptomatic psychotherapy.

39   The relationship between symptomatic therapy and deep psychotherapy in speech pathology is explored in C. Van Riper, "Symptomatic Therapy for Stuttering," in *Handbook of Speech Pathology*, ed. L. E. Travis (New York: Appleton-Century-Crofts, Inc., 1957), pp. 878-96.

Generally, when we speak of *psychotherapy*, however, we mean a procedure which does not aim directly at correction of the given disorder, but tries to delve deeper in order to discover and remedy the "basic causes," of which this (speech) disorder is only one symptom. Further, we mean a psychotherapy which tries to change the patient's entire outlook in order that possible resistance against cure can be reduced. Let us say this clearly: with reference to the treatment of *cluttering,* we believe that such psychotherapeutic intervention is of no avail. First, the clutterer's lighthearted approach to the problems of life make psychotherapeutic intervention difficult. Second, we assume that the roots of cluttering lie in his congenital (hereditary) disposition.

A supportive form of psychotherapy through the authoritative approach is sometimes indicated. In this we strongly attempt to convince the clutterer, who is unaware of his speech disorder, that it would be wise for him to exert the necessary effort to correct his problem. This may be accomplished more facilely, however, by dramatically confronting him with his own mistakes, by a tape recording if possible. Permissiveness on the part of the therapist will only foster the characteristic self-permissiveness of the clutterer. He needs no more. It must be understood that these remarks refer only to pure cluttering and should not necessarily be applied to other speech and voice disorders, whether or not they are co-existent with cluttering.

SELF-IMPROVEMENT

We have never observed a confirmed stammerer who was able to correct his own disorder. The rare cases of self-correction reported are generally individuals who have studied the problem and have undergone a period of self-discipline (usually uncontrolled), and then, having "cured" themselves, open schools for stammerers. Their method consists mainly of drills similar to those that we use in the treatment for cluttering. One might well wonder whether their self-correction claims are reliable, since other claims of theirs are often of doubtful validity. For instance, we know of speech therapists who encourage their patients by informing them that they themselves are former stammerers, although in fact they have experienced no speech problem. Also, we often hear in a case history that a member of the family "was a stutterer and outgrew it." These, however, are generally found to have been clutterers or, at most, clutterer-stammerers.

Many clutterers, on the other hand, especially in families where cluttering is prevalent, learn spontaneously to control their disposition to irregularity of delivery, excess speed, and flagging attention. They become, then, what we call *subclinical clutterers*. For example, I observed a woman, well spoken and versed in several languages, who occasionally exhibited two traits which I assumed to be symptomatic of cluttering. She was a poor teller of jokes and she was unable to render a coherent account of a given event. On approaching the Delaware Memorial Bridge she became fascinated by the name, but was unable to pronounce it: "Delaware Memrial—no—Delaware Momorial—no—Delaware Menemorial—no Delamare. . . ." At this point I interrupted and asked her not to try it again lest she precipitate a phobic reaction. She was particularly disturbed by the repetition of *m*'s in two consecutive syllables. I discovered later on examination that the same difficulty occurred when *m* and *n* followed each other. Thus *antinomy* became *antimonomy, patrimony* became *patrimonomy,* and *ignominy* became *ignomonomy.* In other respects she was a compulsively orderly and organized person, whose attention lapsed only very occasionally, indicating the great effort she exerted to overcompensate for her basic disposition. When particularly interested in what she was saying she might begin a sentence with "I, I, I . . . ," sometimes repeating the pronoun as many as eight or ten times before continuing. She was frightened of public speaking (a symptom typical of cluttering), although preparing for a teaching career. In general she was unaware of her mistakes.

This case is characteristic of many self-improved clutterers. Where effort at self-correction proves insufficient they continue to manifest typical symptoms, and at the same time they become compulsively rigid in those areas which they are able to control successfully. K. de Hirsch [4] also notes compulsive rigidity as a means of self-correction.

When a "stutterer" is able to "outgrow" his disorder, our bias is to assume that he was actually a clutterer, either clinical or subclinical. Often the father of a son in treatment for cluttering or stammering reports that he himself has "outgrown" his "stuttering." We can deduce, however, that the father, having brought his son for treatment, has little or no confidence in the possibility of spontaneous recovery.

In cluttering the chances for self-improvement are tenuous. Most important is that the typical clutterer is unaware of his problem. There seem to be two crucial points at which self-improvement is most likely. These are at the beginning of formal education and at puberty, at which times children must exercise increased self-control over their shortcomings in general. It is at these very times that many clutterers become stammerers, indicating, we believe, that the attempt to overcome cluttering was misdirected. The possibility of self-im-

40   A review of the following book in this context will prove most interesting: W. Johnson, "Study of the Onset and Development of Stuttering," in *Stuttering Children and Adults*, ed. W. Johnson (Minneapolis, Minn.: University of Minnesota Press, 1955), pp. 37-73.

provement in an intelligent and ambitious clutterer does exist, however, when the symptoms are not too difficult to control. Parents should be informed of the necessary prophylactic measures. ᔑᔑᔑ

4 Symposium on Stuttering and Cluttering, New York Society for Speech and Voice Therapy, May 1, 1963.

THE PROGNOSIS FOR CLUTTERING HAS RANGED FROM GOOD TO HOPE-
less. Early investigators, such as E. Colombat (*43*), M. Colombat
(*44*), and Hunt (*103*), wrote that with therapy over a period
of six months to a year the prognosis is good. Gutzmann (*92*)
believed that three to four months of therapy would be sufficient. However, all of these authors are thought to have had
limited experience with cluttering. Liebmann (*119*) apparently
had the most experience, and he indicates that successful treatment requires about one year.

In the first decades of the twentieth century, speech therapists

6 *prognosis and prophylaxis*

found that there was little transference of the control acquired
in therapy to the clutterer's day-to-day performance, and that
relapse was frequent. Accordingly, mention of prognosis disappeared from the literature, but in discussions with colleagues
one heard over and over again that treatment for cluttering
was virtually hopeless. Recently the prognosis has come to be
regarded as rather hopeful, but few authors venture a firm pre-
diction. In our experience with the procedures described in
the preceding chapters we have found that the average intelligent and cooperative patient between the ages of ten and
eighteen requires about one year for successful therapy. They
are seen for half-hour sessions three times a week for the first
four to six months, then twice a week, and finally once a week.
At the conclusion of therapy there is a control period of six
months during which we see the patient once a month. This

schedule is recommended for only those children who are capable of functioning within a school program, although many of them are underachievers. (Academic performance improves as therapy progresses.)

Our experience with older patients and with cases of Central Language Imbalance severe enough to preclude any academic achievement has been insufficient to permit us to evaluate the prognosis for these individuals. Seeman (190) writes that in these cases the prognosis depends upon intelligence, character, and behavior. For example, in cases of "hyperactive" and "nervous" clutterers it is more difficult for the therapist to influence the patient, and accordingly, prognosis is poor. Also, prognosis worsens with increased neuropathological symptomatology (symptomatical cluttering). The attitude and quality of speech of the patient's family is also an important factor. An uncooperative family can compromise the results of the most successful therapy. Luchsinger (126) notes that often one or both parents manifest cluttering symptoms, in which case they should also be given therapy, or at least instruction.

In cases of mild cluttering in children of six to eight years some self-correction can be expected if the parents are informed and cooperative. In these cases we see the child once every six months and advise the parents of the most effective procedures for their specific problem. A typical case is that of a seven-year-old boy whose speech was somewhat rapid and slightly slurred. The parents' report was that he had begun to "stutter." It happened that we knew the family and could point out that the boy's older sister "out-talked" him constantly and that the parents were somewhat impatient. The boy was in a situation where it was almost impossible for him to introduce a thought into the conversation around him. We suggested strict conversational discipline. When one person spoke, no other person was permitted to interrupt. Thus everyone was assured the opportunity of voicing his thoughts, regardless of the time it took. After four weeks the mother reported that the boy's "stuttering" had disappeared completely.

On the whole, then, with proper therapy, prognosis in the average case of cluttering is good. The basic imbalance can be compensated for, although not cured, and concentration of attention is always necessary to maintain the new balance. As therapy progresses, concentration becomes easier for the clutterer, but he will manifest his original symptoms when he is too tired or distracted to concentrate attention on his speech process. Public speaking remains difficult for even the most successfully treated clutterers.

PROPHYLAXIS

The prevention of cluttering has two objectives: (*a*) to prevent cluttering completely or the progression of existing cluttering and (*b*) to prevent conversion of cluttering to stammering.

The basic prophylactic measure is slow and clear speech in the presence of the child. Children learn to speak by imitation,

41   Sound advice is given in C. Van Riper, *Teaching Your Child to Talk* (New York: Harper & Row, Publishers, Inc., 1950).

and it is essential, therefore, that they model their own speech on correct pronunciation, grammar, and sentence structure, as well as on logically constructed accounts. Although a young child cannot master the principles of grammar as such, he will adopt correct usage if that is what he hears.

A more specific measure is to read or tell a short story slowly and clearly to the child, and then have him repeat the story—sentence by sentence. This is of value in acquiring a vocabulary, grammatical sense, and a feeling for general organization—all of which are lacking to some degree in clutterers. In cluttering there is omission of details that are essential to a logically progressive story or account. As a preventive, when the child repeats a story he should be encouraged to include as many details as possible, commensurate with his age and ability. Using psychological terminology, we would say that the clutterer's communicative processes are unstructured, and prophylaxis, therefore, must include insistence on concrete structure as a basis for communication. This should be done as a game, rather than as a task. Pressure or discipline in an attempt to evoke more detail than the child is able to recall with reasonable facility may cause him to add fanciful elements to the story to satisfy the parent. A child's sense of the line between fact and fancy is not as real as an adult's, and in prophylaxis for cluttering the goal is observation and recall of fact. This procedure may appear to limit development and expression of imagination, while the clutterer suffers from too much. In fact, imagination does not develop through a child's contact with adults, but through play with his peers or alone. At most, the adult will forego his pleasure at typical childlike expressions and distortions, but he will be rewarded with adequate communicative processes in his maturing child.

Concentration on detail will be an important factor when children begin to learn to read and write. We cannot embark here on a discussion of the global versus analytic-synthetic reading methods. Specifically in relation to clutterers, however, we insist on the analytic approach. A child with Central Language Imbalance tends to perform all tasks quickly and superficially, disregarding detail. The global approach to reading reinforces his cluttering tendency by stressing consideration of the whole word or phrase rather than the analysis of its component letters and syllables. The result is poor reading and spelling, and sometimes even inability to master all the letters of the alphabet. If a child with Central Language Imbalance is to develop adequate reading and writing skill, teaching of these skills must begin with rigorous analysis of letters and then proceed to syllables and words.

One danger inherent in persistent correction of a child's speech is the possibility that stammering may develop as a result. As we have seen, stammering is a likely outgrowth of cluttering. Age is a significant factor in this regard. The inception of stammering occurs most often between the ages of two and four, at six (concurrent with the beginning of formalized education), and less often at the beginning of puberty. Since stammering can also occur as a result of constant misdirected attempts at correction of speech, parents should not label a child a "stutterer" or insist on repetition of troublesome words or phrases, especially at these sensitive ages. The question might arise as to whether or not the prophylactic measures suggested here might precipitate stammering in a young child. The answer will be negative if two general rules are applied. First, correction should be made positively and pleasantly, never punitively or impatiently. Second, explicit directions should be given when necessary so that the child will not attempt self-correction, which is apt to lead him into further difficulty.

CLUTTERING HAS NOT BEEN MENTIONED IN MOST OF THE AMER-
ican literature on speech pathology. Even in the international
literature, where it has long been considered as a distinct speech
disorder, cluttering has been awarded little importance, either
statistically or pathologically. The assumption that the statistical incidence of cluttering is low is attributed to the clutterers'
lack of awareness of their disorder and to their not seeking
professional help generally. In fact, the incidence of cluttering
is thought to be at least as high as that of stammering.

Cluttering is psychologically significant because it indicates
a general disorder of the language and communication processes. Hence it is usually found in conjunction with problems in

7 *summary*

reading, writing, and musicality, as well as other disorders of
speech and voice. The basic disorder of which cluttering is the
verbal manifestation is called Central Language Imbalance.
There is no evidence of neurological involvement in Central
Language Imbalance, but all indications point to a hereditary
factor. When the characteristic symptoms of cluttering are manifested in cases of neurological lesions, the disorder is called
symptomatic cluttering to distinguish it from typical cluttering.
The severity of the given symptoms varies in individual cases.
Clutterers are quick and superficial in other areas too, and
generally hyperactive and restless. Their disorderliness and
inability to concentrate might imply that clutterers are un-
intelligent, but intelligence is not a major factor, and their
tendency to approach all tasks from a general or global stand-
point can make them especially adept at abstract reasoning.

Psychologically, clutterers demonstrate characteristics which on first encounter might be taken as signs of emotional disturbance. However, careful examination will indicate that these characteristics are rooted in the basic disposition. Clutterers are carefree and impatient, but have a relatively high frustration tolerance. Only when their inability to concentrate becomes a cause of repeated failure (usually in school) are they apt to become explosive and difficult to manage.

Mild cluttering can be self-corrected, but this usually results in rigid compulsiveness in some area of activity, with the basic tendency to disorderliness expressed in other areas. The primary aims of therapy are to increase the ability to concentrate and to direct attention to the details of a task, especially speaking and reading. There are specific exercises geared to correct each symptom. The patient's cooperation and willingness to persist are prerequisites for successful therapy. Without determined effort a clutterer will revert to his natural speech habits when tired or distracted.

Stammering is an outgrowth of cluttering. Therapy for stammering should include treatment of the cluttering component. The interrelationship of cluttering and stammering explains the efficacy of therapeutic measures which heretofore seemed contradictory in purpose.

THIS TEXT PRESENTS A NEW FRAME OF REFERENCE FROM WHICH to view certain theories and clinical practices in the field of speech pathology. Some of these theories and techniques have remained unquestioned for centuries, and accordingly, it is to be expected that many concepts set forth here will meet with resistance. These concepts have been discussed with some of our most experienced colleagues, some of whom vigorously dissented at first. However, many concurred later, after reappraising their own clinical observations.

These theories were not derived from a preconceived hypothesis for which proof was secured a posteriori by specially constructed tests or experiments. On the contrary, they were

epilogue

derived over a period of many years of clinical and therapeutic observation. Preconceived theory is apt to blind an investigator to the realities of clinical observation. However, we consider no clinical observation complete (in the scientific sense) until the case has been dealt with therapeutically.

The emphasis here is on treatment, in compliance with our obligation to patients and because therapeutic experience yields decisive information on the etiology, inner mechanism, and general evaluation of a speech disorder.

One of our most intricate problems was delimitation of Central Language Imbalance and its verbal manifestation, cluttering. Criteria that are too broad would dilute the outlines of the entities and weaken the therapist's grip on the clinical situation. Until now the criteria have been too narrow, and as a result the implications of the common underlying pathology of related language and communication disorders have been overlooked. The criteria established here are more in accord with our clinical and therapeutic experience.

Cluttering is only now beginning to receive the attention it deserves in the literature on speech pathology and in the practice of speech therapy. One of the most important developments in the last decades is recognition by an increasing number of therapists that cluttering has a close and intricate relationship with certain other language disorders, the most important of which are stammering, dyslexia, and dysgraphia.

Cluttering has come of age. ᲽᲽᲽ

bibliography

1. Aetius, Amidensis, *The Four Books of Classical Medicine*. . . . (Lugduni: G. & M. Berings, 1549). In Latin.
2. Anderson, V. A., "The Auditory Memory Span for Speech Sounds," *Speech Monographs*, V (1938), 115-29.
3. Aristotle, *Problems*, trans. W. S. Hett (Cambridge, Mass.: Harvard University Press, 1936).
4. Arnold, G. E., in Luchsinger and Arnold: *Textbook of Voice and Speech Pathology* (Vienna: Springer-Verlag, 1949). In German.
5. ———, in Luchsinger and Arnold: *Textbook of Voice and Speech Pathology*, 2nd ed. (Vienna: Springer-Verlag, 1959). In German.
6. ———, "Studies in Tachyphemia: I. Present Concepts of Etiologic Factors," *Logos*, III (1960).
7. ———, "Studies in Tachyphemia: III. Signs and Symptoms, *Logos*, III (1960).
8. ———, "The Genetic Background of Developmental Language Disorders," *Folia Phoniatrica*, XIII (1961).

9. Arnold, G. E., "Language Disability," *Speech Pathology and Therapy*, VI (1963).

10. Artley, A. Sterl, "A Study of Certain Factors Presumed to Be Associated with Reading and Speech Difficulties," *Journal of Speech and Hearing Disorders*, XIII (1948).

11. Bakwin, K. M. and H. Bakwin, "Cluttering," in *Clinical Management of Behavior Disorders in Children*, 2nd ed. (Philadelphia: W. B. Saunders Co., 1960).

12. Ballet, G., *Inner Speech and Aphasia* (Paris: Librairie Felix Alcan, 1888). In French.

13. Bangs, J., *Idiopathic Language Retardation*, Eighth Congress of the International Association of Logopedics and Phoniatrics, Amsterdam, 1950 (Basel: Karger, 1952).

14. Bazin, David, *Speech and Its Disorders* (Basel: 1717). Quoted from Luchsinger (*121*). In Latin.

15. Beebe, H. A., "Auditory Memory Span for Meaningless Syllables," *Journal of Speech Disorders*, IX (1944).

16. Bell, A. M., *Observations on Speech: The Causes and the Cure of Stammering* (Edinburgh: W. P. Kennedy, 1853).

17. Bender, L., "Problems in Conceptualization and Communication in Children with Developmental Alexia," in *Psychopathology of Communication*, eds. P. Hoch and J. Zubin (New York-London: Grune & Stratton, Inc., 1958).

18. Bente, Schoenharl, and Krump, "EEG-Findings in Stutterers. . . .," *Archiv für Ohren-, usw. Heilkunde*, CXXCIX (1956). In German.

19. Bentzen, F., "Sex Ratios in Learning and Behavior Disorders," *American Journal of Orthopsychiatry*, XXXIII (1963).

20. Berkhan, O., *Disturbances of Speech and Writing* (Berlin: A. Hirschwald, 1889). In German.

21. Bilancioni, G., *Voice in Speaking and Singing* (Rome: Pozzi, 1923). In Italian.

22. Blanton, S., "The Voice and the Emotions," *Quarterly Journal of Public Speaking*, I (1915).

23. Bloodstein, O., "Stuttering as an Anticipatory Struggle Reaction," in *Stuttering*, ed. J. Eisenson (New York: Harper & Row, Publishers, Inc. 1958).

24. ———, "The Development of Stuttering: III. Theoretical and Clinical Implications," *Journal of Speech and Hearing Disorders*, XXVI (1961).

25. Bluemel, C. S., *Stammering and Cognate Defects of Speech* (New York-London-Paris: Stechert-Hafner, Inc., 1913), I and II.
26. ——, *Mental Aspects of Stuttering* (Boston: Williams & Wilkins, 1930).
27. ——, "Primary and Secondary Stammering," *Quarterly Journal of Speech*, XVIII (1932).
28. ——, *The Riddle of Stuttering* (Danville, Ill.: The Interstate Printers and Publishers, 1957).
29. ——, "Concepts of Stammering," *Journal of Speech Disorders*, XXV (1960).
30. Boome, J., "Speech Defects in Young Children," *Public Health* (January, 1937).
31. Borel-Maisonny, S., "Speech Disorders in Dyslectic and Dysorthographic Children," *Enfance*, IV (1951). In French.
32. ——, "Disturbances of Speech Rhythm," in *La Voix* (Paris: Maloine, 1953). In French.
33. Bradford, D., "Studies in Tachyphemia: VII. A Framework of Therapeusis for Articulation Therapy with Tachyphemia and/or General Language Disability," *Logos*, VI (1963).
34. Brickner, R. M., "A Human Cortical Area Producing Repetition," *Journal of Neurophysiology*, III (1940).
35. Brotemarkle, R. A., "Some Memory Span Test Problems," *The Psychological Clinic*, XV (1924).
36. Cabanas, R., "Some Findings in Speech and Voice Therapy among Mentally Deficient Children," *Folia Phoniatrica*, VI (1954).
37. Cadet, C., "Remark on Stuttering," *La médecine éclairée par les sciences physiques*, III (1792). In French.
38. Chervin, Dr., *Stuttering and other functional disorders of speech*, 3rd ed. (Paris: Société d'éditions scientifiques, 1902). In French.
39. Chesni, Y., and F. Kocher, "Comparison of Speed of Spoken Speech and of Verbal Thought," *Revue de Laryngologie* (Bordeaux), LXXIX (1958). In French.
40. Clark, A. S., "Correlation of Auditory Digit Memory Span with Intelligence," *The Psychological Clinic*, XV (1923).
41. Clouston, T. S., *The Neuroses of Development* (Edinburgh: Oliver & Boyd, Ltd., 1891).
42. Coen, R., *Pathology and Therapy of Speech Disturbances* (Vienna-Leipzig: Urban & Schwarzenberg, 1886). In German.

43. Colombat, E., *Textbook of Orthophonics* (Paris: Asselin et Hongeau, 1887). In French.
44. Colombat, M. (de l'Isère), *Stuttering and Other Speech Defects* (Paris: Mansut fils, 1830). In French.
45. Cotton, J. C., "Syllabic Rate: A New Concept in the Study of Speech Rate Variation," *Speech Monographs*, III (1936).
46. Davis, D. M., "The Relation of Repetitions in the Speech of Young Children to Certain Measures of Language Maturity and Situational Factors," Part I, *Journal of Speech Disorders*, IV (1939); Part II, *Idem*, V (1940); Part III, *Idem*, V (1940).
47. Davis H., "Interpretation of the Electrical Activity of the Brain," *American Journal of Psychiatry*, XCIV (1938).
48. De Hirsch, K., "Specific Dyslexia or Strephosymbolia," *Folia Phoniatrica*, IV (1952).
49. ———, "Gestalt Psychology as Applied to Language Disturbances," *Journal of Nervous and Mental Disorders*, CXX (1954).
50. ———, "Predictions of Future Reading Disabilities in Children with Oral Language Disorders," *Folia Phoniatrica*, VII (1955).
51. ———, "Studies in Tachyphemia: IV. Diagnosis of Developmental Language Disorders," *Logos*, IV (1961).
52. ———, "Two Categories of Learning Difficulties in Adolescents," *American Journal of Orthopsychiatry*, XXXIII (1962).
53. ——— and W. S. Langford, "Clinical Note on Stuttering and Cluttering in Young Children," *Pediatrics*, V (1950).
54. De Quirós, B., "Pathology and Therapy of the Rhythmical Disturbances of Speech," *Revue de Laryngologie* (Bordeaux), LXXVII (1956). In French.
55. Diehl, C. F., *A Compendium of Research and Theory on Stuttering* (Springfield, Ill.: Charles C Thomas, Publisher, 1958).
56. Douglass, L. C., "A Study of Bilaterally Recorded Electroencephalograms of Adult Stutterers," *Journal of Experimental Psychology*, XXXV (1943).
57. Dumke, D. H., G. Heese, W. Kroker, and I. Siems, "About the Symptomatology of Cluttering," *Folia Phoniatrica*, XV (1963). In German.
58. Eames, T., "The Relationship of Reading and Speech Difficulties," *Journal of Educational Psychology*, XLI (1950).
59. Eisenson, J., *The Psychology of Speech* (New York: Appleton-Century-Crofts, Inc., 1938).
60. ———, "A Perseveration Theory of Stuttering," in *Stuttering*, ed. J. Eisenson (New York: Harper & Row, Publishers, Inc., 1958).

61. —— and R. Pastel, "A Study of Perseverating Tendency in Stutterers," *Quarterly Journal of Speech,* XXII (1936).

62. Eustis, R. S., "The Primary Etiology of the Specific Language Disabilities," *Journal of Pediatrics,* XXXI (1947).

63. Fairbanks, G. and D. S. Spriesterbach, "A Study of Minor Organic Deviations in "Functional" Disorders of Articulation. I. Rate of Movement of Oral Structures," *Journal of Speech Disorders,* XV (1950).

64. Falck, F. J. and V. T. Falck, "Disorders of Neurological Integrative Mechanisms—A Rationale for the Expansion of Our Professional Scope, *"Journal of American Speech and Hearing Association,* IV (1962).

65. Ferreri, G., "Bibliographical Contributions to Voice and Speech Pathology," *Archivio Italiano di Otologia,* XLIV (1933). In Italian.

66. Fischer, M. S., "Correlation between Repetition and Chronological Age," *Journal of Experimental Education,* I (1932).

67. Flatau, T. S., "Clinical Observations on Stuttering," *Medizinische Welt,* III (1929). In German.

68. Florensky, J. A., "The Problem of Functional Disorders of Speech (Paraphrasia and Tachylalia)," *Zeitschrift für die gesamte Neurologie und Psychiatrie,* CXLVIII (1933). In German.

69. Freund, H., "Personality and Speech Disturbances," *Medizinische Welt,* XXXV (1932). In German.

70. ——, "Relationship between Stuttering and Cluttering," *Monatsschrift für Ohrenheilkunde,* LXVIII (1934). In German.

71. ——, "Studies in the Interrelationship between Stuttering and Cluttering," *Folia Phoniatrica,* IV (1952).

72. Frischeisen-Koehler, I., *The individual speed* (Stuttgart: Georg Thieme Verlag, 1933). In German.

73. Froeschels, E., *Children's Speech and Aphasia* (Berlin: Springer-Verlag, 1918). In German.

74. ——, "The Paragrammatism of Children," *Wiener Medizinische Wochenschrift,* XXXV (1930). In German.

75. ——, *Textbook of Speech Disturbances* (Vienna: F. Deuticke, 1931). In German.

76. ——, "Problem of Cluttering and Stammering," *Wiener klinische Wochenschrift,* L (1937). In German.

77. ——, "Cluttering," *Journal of Speech Disorders,* XI (1946).

78. ——, "The Significance of Symptomatology for the Under-

standing of the Essence of Stuttering," *Folia Phoniatrica,* IV (1952).

79. Froeschels, E., "Contribution to the Relationship between Stuttering and Cluttering," *Logopédie en Phoniatrie,* XXVII, No. 4 (1955).

80. —— and A. Jellinek, "The Importance of Imagery Types in Speaking and Singing," *Wiener medizinische Wochenschrift,* LXXVIII (1928). In German.

81. —— and L. Kallen, "Types of Imagery in Clutterers," *Wiener medizinische Wochenschrift,* XXXV (1930). In German.

82. —— and G. Simon, "Therapeutic Experiences with Speech Disturbances," *Monatsschrift für Ohrenheilkunde,* XLV (1911). In German.

83. Gedda, L., L. Braconi, and G. Bruno, "Stuttering in Twins. . . ." *Acta Geneticae Medicae et Gemellologiae,* IX (1960). In Italian.

84. Gerstman, F. and P. Schilder, "Motor Disturbances," *Zeitschr. f. d. ges. Neurologie u. Psychiatrie,* LXXXVI (1923). In German.

85. Glasner, P. J. and F. S. Vermilyea, "An Investigation of the Definition and Use of the Diagnosis 'Primary Stuttering.' " *Journal of Speech and Hearing Disorders,* XVIII (1953).

86. Goldstein, K., *Language and Language Disturbances* (New York: Grune & Stratton, Inc., 1948).

87. Greene, J. S., "Agitophasia Associated with Agitographia," *Medical Record* (October 28, 1916).

88. —— and E. J. Weil, *The Cause and Cure of Speech Disorders* (New York: The Macmillan Company, 1926).

89. Guiot, C., E. Hertzog, P. Rondot, and P. Molina, "Arrest or Acceleration of Speech Evoked by Thalamic Stimulation in the Course of Stereotaxic Procedures for Parkinsonism," *Brain,* LXXXIV (1961).

90. Guthrie, L. G., *Functional Nervous Disorders in Childhood* (New York: Harcourt, Brace & World, 1907).

91. Gutzmann, H., Sr., *Lectures on Speech Disturbances* (Berlin: S. Fischer, 1893). In German.

92. ——, "Cluttering," in *Speech Pathology,* 3rd ed. (Berlin: S. Fischer, 1924). In German.

93. Gutzmann, H., Jr., "Experiments with Treatment of Speech Disorders with Glutamic Acid," *Folia Phoniatrica,* VI (1954). In German.

94. Haase, C. A., *Stuttering* (Berlin: A. Hirschwald, 1846). In German.
95. Hahn, E. F., *Stuttering; Significant Theories and Therapies,* 2nd ed. (Stanford, Calif.: Stanford University Press, 1956).
96. Hallgren, B., "Specific Dyslexia ('Congenital Word-Blindness')," *Acta Psychologica et Neurologica,* Supplement 65, Stockholm (1950).
97. Hanley, T. D. and W. L. Thurman, *Developing Vocal Skills* (New York: Holt, Rinehart and Winston, Inc., 1962).
98. Hartwell, N. and E. Scarbrough, "A Quantitative and Qualitative Analysis of the Electroencephalograms of Stutterers and Non-Stutterers," *Journal of Experimental Psychology,* XXXII (1943).
99. Hippokrates, *Praecepta* 6, *Aphorisms* 6, 32, *Epidemics* 2, 5 and 2, 6, *De judicatione* 6.
100, Hoepfner, T., "About Stuttering (Associative Aphasia)," *Archiv für Psychiatrie,* LXX (1924). In German.
101. Holst, H., "Demosthenes' Speech Impediment," *Symbolae Osloenses,* fasc. 4, Oslo (1926).
102. Hudson-Makuen, G., "Defects of Speech: Nomenclature," *Laryngoscope,* XX (1910).
103. Hunt, J., *Stammering and Stuttering; their Nature and Treatment,* 7th ed. (London: Longmans, Green & Co., Ltd., 1870). 1st ed. 1861.
104. Istenes, K., "Twenty-five Years of State Courses for the Treatment of Speech Disorders," Budapest: 1925. In Hungarian.
105. Johnson, W., ed. *Stuttering in Children and Adults* (Minneapolis: University of Minnesota Press, 1955).
106. Kagen, B., "Retarded Speech, Alexia and Agraphia....," in *La Voix,* eds. Aubin and Tarneaud (Paris: Maloine, 1953). In French.
107. Kaiser, L., "The Sounds of Speech....,"in *La Voix,* eds. Aubin and Tarneaud (Paris: Maloine, 1953). In French.
108. Kanizsai, D., "The Treatment of Stuttering," *Magyar Gyógypedagógiai Tanárok Közlönye,* 1944. In Hungarian.
109. ———, *Prophylaxis of Speech Disturbances* (Budapest: Tankönyvkiadó, 1954). In Hungarian.
110. Karlin, I. W. and L. Kennedy, "Delay in the Development of Speech," *American Journal of Diseases of Childhood,* LI (1936).
111. Kelly, J. C. and M. D. Steer, "Revised concept of rate," *Journal of Speech and Hearing Disorders,* XIV (1949).

112. King, P. T., "Perseverative Factors in a Stuttering and a Non-Stuttering Population," *Pennsylvania State Review of Educational Research,* V (1953).
113. ——, "Perseveration in Stutterers and Nonstutterers," *Journal of Speech and Hearing Research,* IV (1961).
114. Klencke, P., *The Cure of Stuttering....,*" (Leipzig: Chr. Ernst Rothmann, 1860). In German.
115. Koukol and Poray-Kochitz, "Cluttering....," *Revue française de phoniatrie,* III (1935). In French.
116. Kussmaul, A., "Speech disorders," in *Cyclopedia of the Practice of Medicine* (New York: William Wood & Co., 1877), XIV.
117. Lee, B. S., "Some Effects of Side-Tone Delay," *Journal of the Acoustical Society of America,* XXII (1950).
118. ——, "Effects of Delayed Speech Feedback," *Journal of the Acoustical Society of America,* XXII (1950).
119. Liebmann, A., *Cluttering (Paraphrasia Praeceps),* fasc. 4 of the Lectures on Speech Disturbances (Berlin: O. Coblentz, 1900). In German.
120. ——, "Cluttering (Paraphrasia Praeceps)," *Zeitschrift für die gesamte Neurologie und Psychiatrie,* CXXVII (1930). In German.
121. Luchsinger, R., "Remarks to the History of Phoniatrics in the Eighteenth Century," *Folia Phoniatrica,* III (1951). In German.
122. ——, "Heredity in Speech and Voice Disturbances," *Folia Phoniatrica,* XI (1959). In German.
123. ——, "Stammering," *Phonetica,* III (1959). In German.
124. ——, "Speech Development in Twins and Heredity....," *Folia Phoniatrica,* XIII (1961). In German.
125. ——, "Interverbal and Intraverbal Acceleration in Cluttering. ...," *Archiv für Ohren-Nasen-Kehlkopfheilkunde,* CLXXX (1962). In German.
126. ——, *Cluttering; Diagnosis, Etiology, and Treatment* (Berlin-Charlottenburg: C. Marhold, 1963). In German.
127. —— and R. Brunner, "Investigations of the Speech of Epileptics....," *Folia Phoniatrica,* II (1950). In German.
128. —— and C. Dubois, "Speech Melody in Normal and Stuttering Individuals....," *Folia Phoniatrica,* XV (1963). In German.
129. —— and H. Landolt, 'EEG Investigations in Stammering and Cluttering....," *Folia Phoniatrica,* III (1951). In German.
130. —— and H. Landolt, "Cluttering and Cluttering-Stammering....," *Folia Phoniatrica,* VII (1955). In German.

131. McCall, E., "Two Cases of Congenital Aphasia in Children," *British Medical Journal*, I (1911).

132. McCarthy, D., "Language Development in Children," in Carmichael's *Manual of Child Psychology* (New York: John Wiley & Sons, Inc., 1946).

133. McCauley, S., "A Study of the Relative Value of the Audio-Vocal Forward Memory Span and the Reverse Span as Diagnostic Tests," *The Phychological Clinic*, XVI (1925).

134. McCready, E. B., "Defects in the Zone of Language (Word-Deafness and Word-Blindness) and Their Influence in Education and Behavior," *American Journal of Psychiatry*, VI (1926).

135. Magendie, "Stuttering," in *Dictionnaire de médecine et de chirurgie pratique*, IV (1830). In French.

136. Marland, P., "Shadowing—a Contribution to the Treatment of Stammering," *Folia Phoniatrica*, IX (1957).

137. Meltzer, H., "Personality Differences between Stuttering and Non-Stuttering Children as Indicated by the Rohrschach Test," *Journal of Psychology*, XVII (1944).

138. Mercurialis, H., *Diseases of Children* (Waldkirch: Pernea, 1584). In Latin.

139. Metraux, R. W., "Auditory Memory Span for Speech Sounds of Speech Defective Children Compared with Normal Children," *Journal of Speech Disorders*, VII (1942).

140. Meyer-Eppler, W. and R. Luchsinger, "The Lee Effect in Speech," *Folia Phoniatrica*, VII (1955). In German.

141. Milisen, R., "The Incidence of Speech Disorders," in *Handbook of Speech Pathology*, ed. L. Travis (New York: Appleton-Century-Crofts, Inc., 1957).

142. Moolenaar-Bijl, A., "Therapy of cluttering," *Tijdschrift for Logopedie en Phoniatrie*. In Dutch.

143. ———, "Cluttering (Paraphrasia Praeceps)," in *Twentieth Century Speech and Voice Correction*, ed. E. Froeschels (New York: Philosophical Library, Inc., 1948).

144. Moore, C. A., "Reading and Arithmetic Ability Associated with Speech Defects," *Journal of Speech Disorders*, XII (1947).

145. Morávek, M. and J. Langová, "Some Electrophysiological Findings among Stutterers and Clutterers," *Folia Phoniatrica*, XIV (1962).

146. Morley, M. E., *The Development and Disorder of Speech in Childhood* (Edinburgh and London: E. S. Livingstone Ltd., 1957).

147. Mottier, G., "Speech in children with reading disorders," *Folia Phoniatrica*, III (1951). In German.

148. Nadoleczny, M., "Disorders of Speech and Phonation in Childhood," in *The Diseases of Children*, eds. Pfaundler and Schlossmann (Philadelphia and London: J. B. Lippincott, 1914), V/7.

149. ———, "Cluttering," in *Handbook of Oto-Rhino-Laryngology*, eds. Denker and Kahler (Berlin: Springer-Verlag, 1929), V. In German.

150. ———, "Impediments of Speech Development," *Kinderaerztliche Praxis*, V (1943). In German.

151. Nissim, J., "Speech Disturbances in Neurotics," *Gazette des hôpitaux de Paris*, LXVIII (1895). In French.

152. Ogilvie, M., *Terminology and Definitions of Speech Defects* (New York: Teachers' College, Columbia University, 1942).

153. Orton, S. T., *Reading, Writing and Speech Problems in Children* (New York: W. W. Norton & Company, Inc., 1937).

154. Otto, F., "Speech and Voice Disturbances and the Pfister Test. . . .," *Folia Phoniatrica*, VI (1954). In German.

155. Peacher, W. G., "Neurological Factors in the Etiology of Delayed Speech," *Journal of Speech and Hearing Disorders*, XIV (1949).

156. Pearson, L., "Studies in Tachyphemia: V. Rhythm and Dysrhythmia in Cluttering Associated with Congenital Language Disability," *Logos*, V (1962), 51-59.

157. Perelló, J., "Voice Disturbances and Brain Trauma. . . .," *Revue de Laryngologie* (Bordeaux), LXXXII (1962). In French.

158. Pfaendler, N., "The Geneticist's View of Speech Defects," in *Problèmes actuels de Phoniatrie et de Logopédie*, Supplement No. 1 of *Folia Phoniatrica* (1960). In French.

159. Pichon, E. and S. Borel-Maisonny, "*Stuttering.* . . .," (Paris: Masson et Cie, 1937). In French.

160. ———, and ———, "Psychophysiology of Speech," *Folia Phoniatrica*, I (1948). In French.

161. Pick, A., "The Pathological Disturbances of Expression," *Archives internationales de neurologie*, I, 9th series, 33d year (1911). In French.

162. Plutarch, *The Lives of the Noble Grecians and Romans*, trans. John Dryden (New York: Modern Library, Inc., 1932).

163. Poett, Joseph, Sr., *Practical Treatise on Stammering and Nervous Affections of Speech*, 4th ed. (London: Calbin & Budd, 1833).

164. Poetzl, O., "Physiology and Pathology of the Speed of the Individual," *Wiener klinische Wochenschrift,* LII (1939). In German.

165. Pollak, E. and Schilder, P., "Speech Drive....," *Zeitschrift für die gesamte Neurologie und Psychiatrie,* CIV (1926). In German.

166. Pommez, J., "Remarks on the Treatment of Stuttering," *Revue de Laryngologie* (Bordeaux), LXXIX (1958). In French.

167. Potter, S. O., *Speech and Its Defects* (New York: McGraw-Hill Book Company, 1882).

168. Prescott, D. A., "The Determination of Anatomical Age in School Children and Its Relation to Mental Development," *Harvard Monographs in Education,* Ser. 1, No. 5 (1923).

169. Richter, E, and G. Reuter, "Self-control in Stuttering....," *Die Sprachheilarbeit,* VI (1961). In German.

170. Rieber, R. W., "A Psychological Investigation of the Relationship between Stuttering and Cluttering (Preliminary Report)," *Folia Phoniatrica,* XV (1963).

171. Robbins, S. D., "A New Objective Test for Verbal Imagery Types," *Psychological Review,* XXVII (1920).

172. ———, "The Relation between the Short Auditory Memory Span Disability and Disorders of Speech," *Laryngoscope,* XLV (1935).

173. ———, "The Role of Rhythm in the Correction of Stammering," *Quarterly Journal of Speech,* XXI (1935).

174. ———, *A Dictionary of Speech Pathology and Therapy* (Cambridge, Mass.: Sci-Art Publishers, 1951).

175. Rogerson, C. H., "Congenital Auditory Imperception (Word-Deafness)," *Guy's Hospital Reports,* LXXXIV (1934).

176. Roman-Goldzieher, K., "Graphology of Stutterers, Dyslalics and Clutterers," *Zeitschrift für Kinderforschung,* XXXV (1928). In German.

177. ———, "Handwriting and Speech," *Logos,* II (1959).

178. ———, "Studies in Tachyphemia VI. The Interrelationship of Graphologic and Oral Aspects of Language Behavior," *Logos,* VI (1963).

179. Rullier, "Hésitation," *Dictionnaire de Médecine* (Paris: Bechet, 1821), III. In French.

180. Saunders, M. L., "The Short Auditory Span Disability," *Childhood Education,* VIII (1931).

181. Schick, A., "Etiologic Aspects of Psychiatric Disorders and Their Implications for Therapy," *American Journal of Psychotherapy*, XXVI (1962).
182. Schilder, P., "Multiple Sources of Psychic Energy....," *Archiv für Psychiatrie*, LXX (1924). In German.
183. ———, "Central Disturbances of Motor Speech....," *Wiener Medizinische Wochenschrift*, LXXVII (1927). In German.
184. Schilling, R., "Inner Language," *Zeitschrift für Psychologie*, CXI (1929). In German.
185. ———, "Inner Language and Speech Development," *Medizinische Klinik*, I (1934). In German.
186. Schuell, H., "Sex Differences in Relation to Stuttering. I," *Journal of Speech Disorders*, XI (1946).
187. Scripture, E. W., *Stuttering and Lisping* (New York: The Macmillan Company, 1912).
188. Sedláčková, E., "Vegetative Balance in Stutterers and Clutterers," *Folia Phoniatrica*, XV (1963). In French.
189. Seeman, M., "Pathogenesis of Stuttering. ...," *La Presse Médicale*, CLIX (1951). In French.
190. ———, *Speech Disorders in Childhood* (Halle a. d. Saale: C. Marhold, 1959). In German.
191. ———, and A. Novak, "Motor Ability in Clutterers," *Folia Phoniatrica*, XV (1963). In German.
192. Serre (d'Uzès), "Gesturing in Stuttering. ...," *Gazette médicale de Paris*, V (1837). In French.
193. Seth, G. and D. Guthrie, *Speech in Children. Its Development and Disorders* (London: Oxford University Press, 1935).
194. Shepherd, G., "Studies in Tachyphemia II. Phonetic Description of Cluttered Speech," *Logos*, III (1960).
195. Spearman, C. E., *The Abilities of Man* (New York: The Macmillan Company, 1927).
196. Stambak, M., "The Problem of Rhythm in the Development of the Child and in the Developmental Dyslexias," *Enfance*, IV (1951). In French.
197. Starr, A. S., "The Diagnostic Value of the Audio-Vocal Memory Span," *The Psychological Clinic*, XV (1923).
198. Steer, M. D., "Symptomatologies of Young Stutterers," *Journal of Speech Disorders*, II (1937).
199. Stojanow, W. and R. Heidrich, "The EEG during Autogenous Training," *Psychiatrie, Neurologie und Medizinische Psychologie*, XIV (1962). In German.

200. Streifler, F. and M. Gumpertz, "Cerebral Potentials in Stuttering and Cluttering," *Confinia Neurologica*, XV (1955).
201. Stulli, L., "Cluttering (1827)," *Archivio italiano di otologia*, XLIV (1933). In Italian.
202. Tanner, J. M., *Education and Physical Growth* (London: University of London Press, 1961).
203. Tiffin, J. and M. D. Steer, "An Experimental Analysis of Emphasis," *Speech Monographs*, IV (1937).
204. Town, C. H., "Congenital Aphasia," *The Psychological Clinic*, V (1911).
205. Travis, L. E., *Speech Pathology* (New York: Appleton-Century-Crofts, Inc., 1931).
206. —— and W. Malamud, "Brain Potentials from Normal Subjects, Stutterers and Schizophrenics," *American Journal of Psychiatry*, XCIII (1937).
207. Treitel, L., "Disturbances of Speech Development....," *Archiv für Psychiatrie*, XXIV (1892).
208. Van Dantzig, B., "Writing, Typewriting, and Speaking," *Tijdschrift van Logopedie en Phoniatrie*, XI, No. 5 (1939). In Dutch.
209. Van Dantzig, M., "Syllable-tapping, a New Method of the Help of Stammerers," *Journal of Speech Disorders*, V (1940).
210. Van Riper, C., "Effect of the Devices for Minimizing Stuttering or the Creation of Symptoms," *Journal of Abnormal and Social Psychology*, XXXII (1937).
211. ——, *Speech Correction*, 3rd and 4th eds. (Englewood Cliffs, N.J.: Prentice-Hall, Inc., 1954 and 1963).
212. Verzeano, M., "Time Patterns of Speech in Normal Subjects," *Journal of Speech and Hearing Disorders*, XV (1950).
213. Voelker, C. H., "Incidence of Pathologic Speech Behavior in the American General Population," *Archives of Otolaryngology*, XXXVIII (1943).
214. ——, "Preliminary Investigation for a Normative Study of Fluency," *American Journal of Orthopsychiatry*, XIV (1944).
215. Weiss, D. A., "Combination of Stuttering and Cluttering. ...," *Mitteilungen aus dem logopaedischen Ambulatorium* (Vienna), II, No. 6 (1934). In German.
216. ——, "Contribution to the Problem of Cluttering....," *Mitteilungen ueber Sprach- und Stimmheilkunde*, I, Nos. 4-5 (1935). In German.
217. ——, "Cluttering and Its Treatment....," *Monatsschrift für Ohrenheilkunde*, LXX (1936). In German.

218. Weiss, D. A., "Organic Lesions Leading to Speech Disorders," *Nervous Child,* VII (1948).
219. ———, "Cluttering. A Basic Analysis." Lecture in the New York Society for Speech and Voice Therapy, February 5, 1950.
220. ———, "The Pubertal Change of the Human Voice (Mutation)," *Folia Phoniatrica,* II (1950).
221. ———, "Relationship between Cluttering and Stammering. . . .," *Folia Phoniatrica,* II (1950). In German.
222. ———, *Stuttering: Significant Theories and Therapies,* 2nd ed., ed. E. F. Hahn (Stanford: Stanford University Press, 1956).
223. ———, "Therapy of Cluttering," *Folia Phoniatrica,* XII (1960).
224. ———, "Logopedic observations in a mental hospital," *Folia Phoniatrica* (in print).
225. ——— and H. Beebe, *The Chewing Approach in Speech and Voice Therapy* (Basel-New York: S. Karger, 1950).
226. West, R., M. Ansberry, and A. Carr, *The Rehabilitation of Speech,* 3rd ed. (New York: Harper & Row, Publishers, Inc., 1957).
227. Weuffen, M., "Testing of Word-Finding in Normal and Stuttering Children . . . . ," *Folia Phoniatrica,* XIII (1961). In German.
228. Widmann, N., "Therapy of an Amnesic Clutterer," *Zeitschrift für Kinderforschung,* XVI (1911). In German.
229. Wingate, M. E., "Evaluation and Stuttering: I. Speech Characteristics of Young Children," *Journal of Speech and Hearing Disorders,* XXVII (1962).
230. Wolf, A. A. and E. G. Wolf, "Feedback Processes in the Theory of Certain Speech Disorders," *Speech Pathology and Therapy,* II (1959).

index

index